ATKINS DIET PLAN 2019-2020

The Ultimate Beginner's Guide and Step by step Simpler Way to Lose Weight (Lose Up to 20 Pounds in 3 Weeks)

EMMA BAKER

COPYRIGHT © 2019 BY EMMA BAKER

All rights reserved.

No part of this book may be reproduced in any form or by any electronic or mechanical means, including information storage and retrieval systems, without written permission from the author, except for the use of brief quotations in a book review.

TABLE OF CONTENTS

- THE ATKINS DIET 1
- THE PRINCIPLE OF ATKINS THE DIET 2
- THE COURSE OF THE ATKINS DIET 3
- ATKINS NUTRITION PLAN FOR PHASE I 6
- RECIPES FOR THE ATKINS DIET PLAN (PHASE 1): 7
- ATKINS DIET 2.0 - SLIMMING FASTER AND MORE EFFECTIVELY . 12
- ATKINS DIET 2.0 - THE KETOGENIC DIET 15
- BENEFITS OF THE KETOGENIC DIET 19
- ATKINS DIET: ALLOWED FOOD 51
- KETOSIS: WHAT WAS THAT EXACTLY AGAIN? 54
- HOW IS THE ATKIN'S DIET DIFFERENT FROM THE KETOGENIC DIET? 56
- DIET OF KETONIC VS. ATKINS 60
- ATKINS RECIPES 62
- FOR WHOM IS THE ATKINS DIET SUITABLE? 106
- HOW INDIVIDUAL IS THE ATKINS DIET? 107
- WHAT DIFFERENTIATES LCHF FROM ATKINS? 114
- THE FAQ ON ATKINS DIET 116
- CONCLUSION 126

THE ATKINS DIET

This diet is named after its inventor Robert Atkins and is based on the low-carb principle, or Robert Atkins is the inventor of this diet model. The Atkins diet offers the advantage that you do not have to starve to lose weight; it just has to be done rigorously without carbohydrates. The menu includes meat, fish, eggs, and dairy products, as well as a small selection of vegetables. The fruit is not in the diet of the Atkins diet because fruit contains fructose, so carbohydrates.

For many people who want to lose weight, the Atkins diet is a good alternative to calorie-restricted diets, as the Atkins diet allows you to eat almost any amount of the permitted food. The principle of the diet is based on the assumption that for the utilization and preparation of fats carbohydrates are needed, these are absent with the food intake, the supplied fat is excreted, and also the fat burning of the body is stimulated.

The Atkins diet sparked a veritable hype in the 1980s and became the food model of the beautiful and famous in Hollywood. Many of today's low-carb diets are based on the Atkins-based principle, but many of the strict rules have been softened and, for example, not so rigorously without fruit. During the Atkins diet, sugar, desserts, pasta such as pasta and bread, as well as most fruit, must be avoided.

THE PRINCIPLE OF ATKINS THE DIET

The Atkins diet allows protein and fat. The human body cannot store the protein, and therefore, excess amounts are eliminated. The fat, in turn, cannot be processed without the carbohydrates.

The Atkins diet is based on the assumption that carbohydrates are needed for the metabolism of fats.

If these are no longer supplied, the fat absorbed by the food can no longer be processed and is excreted. Also, the renunciation of carbohydrates leads to a change in metabolism. Carbohydrates are absorbed quickly into the blood and quickly increase blood sugar levels. By eliminating carbohydrates, the blood sugar level remains constantly low. A low blood sugar level, in turn, stimulates fat burning, which in spite of high fat intake in the Atkins diet leads to the breakdown of the stored fat reserves. This describes the state of ketosis desired in the Atkins diet.

In ketosis, ketone bodies are formed in the blood in the liver to replace the lack of glucose in the blood from the carbohydrates. For such "hunger states," the liver can extract ketone bodies from the fat reserves. So to keep the low blood sugar level at a constant level, the body relies on the processing of fat reserves. Incidentally, the ketone bodies are created in every situation in which the body has to resort to the burning of its fat reserves. A sweetish-acetone-like bad breath can recognize people with ketosis.

THE COURSE OF THE ATKINS DIET

The Atkins diet runs in several phases. In the initial phase of the diet is about the state of ketosis, so to achieve the combustion of their fat reserves by carbohydrate avoidance. Atkins' intake of carbohydrates has to be drastically reduced in this phase. Atkins recommended not consuming more than five grams of carbs a day, but later he withdrew that rigorous amount and allowed a maximum of 20 grams of carbohydrates a day.

Mainly overweight persons should take thereby however fewer carbohydrates, to start the fat burning as fast as possible.

The first and strictest phase of the Atkins diet was to last for several weeks. Meat, eggs, fish, cheese, and other dairy products are allowed in a sufficient amount of saturation. Atkins himself has criticized the presentation of his diet as an invitation to dine. Atkins himself suggests no large portions, but moderate and satisfying amounts, after all, the sense of this unusual diet is indeed decrease without hunger, but gluttony is not meant. Once the condition of fat burning has started without starving, the number of carbohydrates may be increased a little daily, for example, a piece of fruit.

In this **second phase** of the diet, the number of carbohydrates may be increased until the weight loss stagnates. Then the amount must be brought back to the last state, at which still a weight loss has taken place.

This **third phase** is maintained until the desired weight loss occurs. After that, the Atkins diet is by no means over. After reaching his desired weight, you can again daily increase the number of carbohydrates until the weight comes to a standstill. This diet should now be maintained permanently. Atkins himself recommends the additional intake of dietary supplements.

A typical day during the Atkins diet

Since bread is mostly taboo in the Atkins diet, breakfast is unusual for German standards. For example, a typical breakfast in the Atkins diet consists of eggs with ham or even bacon, although it may be two eggs in the pan and the bacon does not have to be lean. Unsweetened coffee or tea is allowed in any amount.

Lunch is usually mainly meat, which may be steak or meatballs. It may be a small portion of low-carbohydrate vegetables, such as broccoli or spinach.

For dinner you could, for example, take fried fish. Also, a cheese platter with associated wine is allowed in the Atkins diet.

If you like to nibble something in between and want to stick to the Atkins diet, you can eat bacon cubes or cheese cubes. Also, an egg in between is allowed.

The benefit of the Atkins diet is that you are allowed to eat your fill during meals and can also take snacks; you just have to stick to the approved food. In this direction, you are not bound to tight diet plans with an Atkins diet and can also eat at all times of the day.

Does this really work - eat and lose weight?

Atkins diet leads to weight loss. The body responds to the little blood sugar level by releasing ketone bodies from the stored fat in the liver to keep the blood sugar level constant. However, the weight loss is not overly high; average subjects lost to a study only about five kilograms within a year. And sticking to the Atkins diet is also not easy because of the lack of carbohydrates. Basic foods such as potatoes or bread are forbidden, and the abandonment of fresh fruit is difficult for many people willing to lose weight.

Criticism of the Atkins diet

The originally highly praised Atkins diet is today very controversial. This is partly due to the very one-sided diet with lots of meat and protein. The lack of fruits and vegetables inevitably leads to deficiency symptoms, so that Atkins himself recommends the intake of supplements in addition to his diet. Even a diet without a varied diet is difficult to endure, even the biggest meat lover, the 23st steak finally hungrily literally. Also, the Atkins diet is recommended only for healthy people, so before starting a visit to the doctor should take place in which the personal cardiovascular situation is checked, and the most important laboratory parameters are determined.

In particular, the kidney values must be in order because the diet for kidney patients may even be dangerous because of the high protein content.

The deliberately induced ketosis can be pointed in the form of ketoacidosis, a hyperacidity of the blood, dangerous. Today, many more balanced diets are known, which use the low-carb approach of Atkins, but allow a higher proportion of fruits and vegetables and which overall allow a gentler treatment of health than the strict Atkins diet. Those who still want to get involved in this diet should not give up the previous visit to the doctor and monitor his laboratory parameters during the diet.

ATKINS NUTRITION PLAN FOR PHASE I

You want to feed yourself at Atkins and are looking for an Atkins diet plan for Phase I? Then you are right here! In Phase I of the Atkins diet, you have to restrict yourself, no question. The aim is to reduce the carbohydrate content per day to a maximum of 20g of carbohydrates at this stage (similar to many other low carb diets). Meat, fish, eggs, cheese, and vegetables (with a maximum carbohydrate content of 10g) are allowed. Of fruits, nuts, grains or sugars are in phase I of the Atkins diet taboo. For vegetables, you can choose between tomatoes, lettuce, cucumber, celery, radishes, peppers, mushrooms, avocado, asparagus, spinach, cauliflower, broccoli, green beans, and eggplant. You should try to eat 3 meals a day. However, if you are hungry between meals, raw food, cheese chips, bacon chips or Gouda cubes (note, not too many!) Are perfect as a snack. Here's our 7-day Atkins Diet Plan for Phase I Atkins Diet:

RECIPES FOR THE ATKINS DIET PLAN (PHASE 1):

Monday, Day 1 of the Atkins Diet:

Breakfast: Let's start with a coffee or herbal tea, 2 hard-boiled eggs (carbohydrates: 2.2g, calories: 310kcal) and 1 pack of Stremel salmon, natural (125g) (carbs: 0.1g, calories: 273) that you get a total of 2.3g carbohydrates and 583 calories at breakfast.

For lunch, there's Caesar's salad with chicken breast fillet. You can prepare it very well and bring it to the office in a fresh box. Just before eating, just give the dressing over it. Finished! At noon we come to 2.6g carbohydrates and 440 calories.

In the evening it should be something warm. We just roast two beef hamburgers. Of course, we only eat the meat, because the rolls and sugary sauces are taboo. Carbohydrates: 0g, calories: 468 kcal. There are 200g of vegetables (from the vegetables above freely selectable, either fresh from the market or the freezer.) We decide today for a zucchini-vegetable-pan from the deep freeze. This beats with 6.4g carbohydrates and 104 calories to book, so the dinner totaled 6.4g carbohydrates and 572 calories.

On Day 1 of the Atkins diet, we bring it to the following values:

Carbohydrates: 11.3 g, calories: 1595 kcal

Tuesday, Day 2 of the Atkins Diet

We start again with our coffee or herbal tea and 3 bacon egg muffins. If you are in a hurry in the morning, you can pack the muffins super and eat on the way to the office. The 3 muffins come to a total of 2.7g carbohydrates and 552 calories.

For lunch, there are meatballs filled with feta cheese. The meatballs bring it to 978.5 calories with 3.9g carbohydrates per serving. If you need something fresh, cut half a snake cucumber into small vegetable sticks and nibble on it. The snake cucumber has only 1.6g of carbs at 12 calories. So we come to a total of 990.5 calories and 5.6g calories at lunch.

In the evening there's a stuffed avocado. However, we leave the balsamic vinegar out of the recipe. It has too much sugar. So the dinner for 2 filled avocado halves stays at a slim 10.8g carbs and 24.4 calories.

On Day 2 of our Atkins diet, we come to the following total values: 19.1g carbs, calories: 1566.9 kcal.

Wednesday, Day 3 of the Atkins Diet

This morning we stir 1 cup (200g) cottage cheese with salt, pepper and a few fresh herbs as desired and eat it together with some raw food. The cottage cheese beats with 206 calories and 5.4g carbohydrates. We cut half a snake cucumber into vegetable sticks. The snake cucumber has only 1.6g of carbs at 12 calories. So the breakfast comes to 7g total carbs and 218 calories.

At lunchtime, there is a delicious Greek salad. If you are on the road, you can order it without problems in the restaurant. Otherwise the salad is great to prepare it. The salad has 7.7g of carbs and 517.2 calories.

For dinner, we treat ourselves to a steak (200g). That beats with 2g carbs and 260g calories. There are 100g Italian pan-fried vegetables from the freezer (carbohydrates: 3.5g, calories: 272). The dinner is 5,5g carbs and 532 calories.

All in all, on Day 3 of the Atkins Diet, we get the following values: 20.2g carbs and 1527.2 calories.

Thursday, day 4 of the Atkins diet

Today's breakfast is hearty egg muffins. However, since we are in Phase 1, we do not give milk to the egg mass. The possibilities of variation are almost inexhaustible. Whether tomatoes, broccoli florets, bacon, spinach, feta or grated cheese the egg muffins are simply delicious and taste warm and cold. We approve 2 egg muffins and come (depending on the variation) in total to 4g carbohydrates and 174 calories.

We prepared for lunch the night before because we have prepared stuffed eggplant. With minced meat and cheese, the dish provides a good saturation and leaves us strengthened in the afternoon. The filled eggplants have 16.4g carbohydrates and 561 calories per serving.

In the evening we let it go well. There is chicken breast fillet with feta tomato sauce. This dish has just 3g of carbohydrates at 223.4 calories.

On Day 4 of the Atkins diet, we come up with the following values: 23.4g carbs, 958.4 calories.

Friday, Day 5 of the Atkins Diet

We start in classic style on Friday. With a quick breakfast classic: bacon and eggs, eggs, bacon, and cherry tomatoes. All in all, we get 5.5 grams of carbs and 366 calories.

At lunchtime, we treat ourselves to a gouda salad. It's best to prepare already on Thursday evening so that you only have to grab Friday morning in the fridge. The Gouda salad has 6.3g and 662.5 calories.

In the evening there are 150g shrimp fried in garlic. The shrimp have an unbelievable 0g carbs and 126 calories. The prawns come with 200g of Asian frozen deep-frozen vegetables, with 68 calories and 9.6g of carbs.

For Day 5 of the Atkins diet, we come up with the following values: 21.4g carbohydrates at 1222.5 calories.

Saturday, day 6 of the Atkins diet

On Saturday it may be a bit more elaborate. Today, there is a delicious leek ham omelet in the morning (by the way, it tastes great too!!!). So we come to breakfast at 4.4g carbohydrates and 493 calories.

For lunch, there are stuffed zucchini. The sate wonderful and just tastes great! Carbohydrates: 7.9g, Calories: 303, 9.

In the evening there is a creamy cauliflower puree (5.4g carbohydrates, 124.5 calories) with minced meat topping. For the minced meat just take 250g of mixed minced meat. Clean onion and a stick of leek and mince it. Fry the onions in a pan, add the minced meat and the puree, sauté it, and then add salt, pepper, and paprika and then pour over the cauliflower purée. The minced meat topping has 0.25g carbs and 336 calories.

All in all, on Day 6 of the Atkins Diet, we get the following: 17.95g carbs, 1257.4 calories.

Sunday, day 7 of the Atkins diet

Sunday starts very comfortably, how it could be otherwise than with a Sunday scrambled an egg. The breakfast beats with 251 calories and 2.6g carbohydrates.

For lunch, we treat ourselves to a salmon fillet on spinach. That's just 2.1g of carbs at 316.8 calories.

On Sundays, you have a bit more time to be in the kitchen. We, therefore, prepare a healthy ratatouille for dinner. Advantage: We take the rest the next day to the office. So we do not have to bother about what we eat tomorrow. The ratatouille has 13.7g of carbohydrates at 906 calories, so on Day 7 of the Atkins Diet we get a total of 18.4 carbohydrates and 1473.8 calories.

ATKINS DIET 2.0 - SLIMMING FASTER AND MORE EFFECTIVELY

So that we can all start from the same level of knowledge, this is a brief summary that core theses and phases of the Atkins diet and explain where the shortcomings of the Atkins diet are and how to improve them.

Phase I (induction diet)

In the introductory phase of the diet, fat burning should be greatly increased, and ketosis should be initiated. In this phase, a maximum of 20 g of carbohydrates is consumed daily. The staple foods in this phase should be lettuce, vegetables, eggs, and meat. Soy is also allowed. This phase lasts 14 days and aims to end up being in the so-called ketosis / ketogenic diet.

Phase II (reduction diet)

At this stage, the carbohydrates are increased by 5g daily per week; the target range should be 40-60g carbohydrates daily. You can eat more vegetables, nuts, berries, seeds, and some beans. Otherwise, much remains the same in comparison to Phase I, just a few more complex carbohydrates. As soon as you notice that you no longer lose weight during weekly weighing, the carbohydrates should be reduced again. The goal in this phase is to lose as much weight as possible.

Phase III (pre-maintenance diet)

This phase is to prepare the maintenance diet; the carbohydrates are increased until you no longer decrease or reached its target weight. The recommended carbohydrate sources are those known from Phase II.

Phase IV (Lifelong Maintenance Diet): The actual diet is over, and you have not been in ketosis for a long time. This phase should be maintained for a lifetime to maintain the target weight. It's a kind of low carb paleo diet, where the main focus is on fruits, vegetables, healthy fats, and meat. Larger carbohydrate sources such as cereals and potatoes should continue to be enjoyed only moderately.

This is how the Atkins diet ends, with groundbreaking successes. Yes, and that's one reason why Atkins is not as successful today as it used to be:

The Atkins diet had some weaknesses - disadvantages of the Atkins diet

Atkins 2.0 no longer has these vulnerabilities. They are the following:

- **TOO MUCH PROTEIN**

One of the basics of the Atkins diet is to keep blood sugar levels as constant as possible while avoiding carbohydrates. But insulin, the hormone that is released by carbohydrates, is also formed by protein consumption (by various protein sources) from the body. Too much protein, therefore, also means too high an insulin level that prevents the condition of ketosis. Ideally, the protein content is much lower than in the Atkins diet.

- **TOO LITTLE FAT**

The condition of ketosis is achieved, especially in less overweight users only if at the same time, low protein and carbohydrate content of the food and the fat content is correspondingly high. The liver needs the signal on dietary fats to form ketones.

- **SOY**

Soy as a legume and as controversial food should not play a role in a disciplined diet such as Atkins or Ketose. The absolute exceptions are vegetarians or vegans who carry out this diet but would also advise this to soy only as an absolute exception.

- **PROBIOTICS**

Today it is known that the intestinal flora makes a significant contribution to metabolic health, and a diseased bowel can be a major problem. The knowledge that was not available in the seventies is today. So probiotics such as yogurt, kombucha or apple cider vinegar should also play an important role.

We have clarified what the Atkins Diet is exactly and why it was and still is very successful, but still has some weak points.

ATKINS DIET 2.0 - THE KETOGENIC DIET

What is the ketogenic diet?

For about five years, the ketogenic diet in Germany has also become popular, but it has always been subject to intense criticism, especially from the public side such as the DGE. This is because the ketogenic diet seems to contradict many common dietary recommendations (very few carbohydrates, a lot of fat). So it does not count as a "balanced diet."

But it does not necessarily have to be a balanced diet because it is not intended for everyone as a longer-term diet. The ketogenic diet was established about 100 years ago for therapeutic purposes: at that time, it was used to treat epileptic children and was very successful.

Over the last 100 years, the ketogenic diet has been used for all sorts of therapeutic purposes, and a whole range of uses has arisen.

Since the body is in ketosis and fat burning mode 24 hours a day and the ketogenic diet offers some compelling benefits, it is very, very good for losing weight (fast losing weight) as a diet. ketogenic means that a condition or food supports the formation of ketone bodies in the liver. This term is also common here.

But where is the difference between both forms of diet?

The differences between the Atkins diet and the ketogenic diet. The direct comparison

Scientific Findings

The Atkins Diet was established in the 1970s and 1980s and has not adapted as much too new scientific insights as it should. The ketogenic diet, however, already. It is built according to the current scientific standard.

Ketosis

The state of ketosis can be achieved more easily by a good ketogenic diet than by Atkins since the protein content is very low and the fat content is very high. It was not always the case with Atkins.

Better Nutrition Plans

The ketogenic diet has learned from apps and reviews, and over time has developed better nutritional plans (and healthier nutritional plans).

Success

The Atkins diet is successful, no question. But the ketogenic diet is more sound and practical in direct comparison.

Low Carb Junk Food

Atkins Inc. has also developed low carb bars over time to make the diet more suitable for everyday use. However, these low-carb foods hide nothing but healthy-selling junk food. The ketogenic diet, however, relies 100% on natural foods.

Disadvantages of ketogenic diet/diet:

Hard change

Since most of our dietary calories are normally based on carbohydrates and these are almost completely omitted, a change is needed. Fat burning needs to be greatly increased, and cravings for carbohydrates greatly reduced. The transition into ketosis takes a few days and requires discipline and perseverance. It is worthwhile, however!

Discipline

Not only does carbohydrate disappear and some sort of carbohydrate deprivation sets in, but also the food choices are limited in the ketogenic diet: typical and familiar foods like pizza, pasta, and bread are left out, and many users are missing something in their daily lives. However, these are all foods that make weight loss enormously difficult so that the discipline will be rewarded.

Fat digestion

Since fat consumption is greatly increased and many are not used to it, some users are sensitive to the large amounts of fat. The digestion must first adapt to this, and it is recommended to carry out a slow change over 2-3 weeks, not overnight, into ketosis.

Halitosis

You notice that you are in ketosis if you have a slightly fruity bad breath. This is because a degradation product of the ketone body is exhaled as acetone and you can smell it. It is recommended to take lots of water and herbal tea and to use sugar-free peppermint sweets and chewing gum. Then nobody realizes it.

Physiological insulin resistance

Since temporarily almost no carbohydrates are consumed, the blood sugar level but constant remains, the body goes into a temporary state of insulin resistance. However, this condition is temporary and has nothing to do with diabetes! Nevertheless, it is recommended to eat a few carbohydrates (from healthy sources, i.e., no cereals, gluten, and sugar) "1-2 weeks" after 1 to 2 weeks of ketogenic feeding. If you stick to it, you have nothing to fear.

Ketogenic diet and diabetes

The ketogenic diet can be a very useful and very effective intervention in type 1 diabetes and type 2 diabetes.

Isocaloric Disadvantages

If you carry out the ketogenic diet without losing weight, isocaloric, then I recommend that you only carry out the ketogenic diet for a maximum of two months. After about 6-8 weeks, the isocaloric ketogenic diet causes a very high blood lipid level. In this case, please use the ketogenic diet only temporarily to take advantage of it. But the benefits are:

BENEFITS OF THE KETOGENIC DIET

100% fat burning

You are 24 hours a day, 100% only burn on fat. A fat-burning machine. Ideal for losing weight and reducing fat and one reason why the ketogenic diet is so successful.

Mental clarity

That you are deep in the ketosis, you realize it also because you are very clear in the head and high brain performance to the day. This is because ketone bodies are a very efficient source of energy for the body, and the brain is more energy-releasing than glucose. You notice this extra energy very much.

Less hunger and appetite

Ketones are appetite-inhibiting; because of the huge fat and fiber consumption you are full for longer, ideal for a diet.

The lower need for sleep

The hormones adapt quite well to ketosis, and two hormones that are responsible for nighttime repair (while you sleep) are elevated in ketosis: GABA and HGH (human growth hormone). Therefore, many users of ketosis are observed to suddenly get by with 1 hour less sleep per night, wake up earlier in the morning, and healthy sleep is generally easier.

Endurance

For endurance sports in the non-maximum intensity range, i.e. Normal jogging, hiking, cycling, or swimming, the body prefers to use fat. In ketosis, this fat burning is more efficient and more than normal, and so also a better endurance in sports is achieved. If endurance sports are used together with ketosis, weight loss is greatly increased.

Higher metabolic rate

The energy consumption of the body is slightly increased for me ketosis Falling blood pressure

In various ways, ketone bodies in the body activate biochemical signals that lower blood pressure.

Rising libido

In men, due to the high-fat consumption, an increased testosterone level and increased libido are often observed. Is ketosis worth trying for you now?

Better mood

As fasting is mimicked, the body releases endorphins and increases serotonln, resulting in an improved mood once you are properly in the ketosis.

LDL cholesterol drops

This is interesting for patients with high cholesterol. In the ketogenic diet (in most diets, but especially in ketosis), the harmful LDL cholesterol decreases.

Antioxidant

Ketones can neutralize free radicals (oxidative stress) by reacting with them themselves, but also activate enzymes in the body that can. Inflammations in the body can be alleviated.

Anti-catabolic

Athletes also benefit from the ketogenic diet because athletes are afraid of losing muscle during the diet. Ketones are highly anti-catabolic, so little to no muscle mass is broken down.

Hypoallergenic

Why is not yet known? But it is clear that allergic reactions in the ketosis are much less, as the immune system seems calmed.

Consumers more aware of carbohydrates through Atkins diet

Thanks to the still popular Atkins diet, consumers are "more carb-conscious," and the number of new low-carb products in Europe has doubled in the last five years. This is according to research from the globally leading research agency Mintel.

According to the researchers, the doubling of the number of products is largely due to the rise of the Atkins diet in 2004. Since then, other low-carb diets and low-carbohydrate foods have generally become increasingly popular. Laura Jones, food analyst at Mintel: "The Atkins diet succeeded in making people more aware of carbohydrates and making consumers think about the quality and quantity of carbohydrates."

Pasta

This year, 10 percent of the new low-carb products consisted of substitutes for pasta. Also, baking ingredients (10 percent), bread (9 percent), and energy bars (8 percent) came on the market.

The countries where most new low carb products were launched are France (accounting for a share of 17 percent), Germany and Spain (15 percent each).

Three times as many protein-rich products

Also, many protein-rich products generally well suited to a low carb diet have been added. Since 2008 it has been almost three times as many products. 24 percent of those products consist of protein-rich snacks, 20 percent of dairy and 15 percent of fish, meat, and egg products.

Low-carbohydrate products have not yet massively conquered the market, but new launches are expected to appeal to an ever-increasing audience.

What if it was all one big lie?

First, they ridicule Robert Atkins, author of the greatest bestseller ever (Dr. Atkins 'Diet Revolution and Dr. Atkins' New Diet Revolution) for 30 years and accuse him of quackery and deception, only to discover that Dr. Atkins has always been right.

Or perhaps it was: they discover that their dietary requirements - "eat less fat and more carbohydrates" are the cause of the ongoing obesity epidemic in America. Or, who knows, they discover that both of the above statements are true.

When Atkins first printed his "Diet Revolution" in 1972, Americans were just getting used to the idea that fat especially the saturated fats from meat and dairy products was the main dietary ghost of the American diet.

Atkins managed to sell millions of books. He promised that we could lose weight by eating steak, eggs, and butter, as much as we wanted. Because it is carbohydrates, pasta, rice, and sugar that create obesity and even cardiovascular disease. Fat, he said, was harmless.

Atkins allowed his readers to eat, as he put it, "unlimited, really luxurious food": "lobster with butter sauce, steak with bearnaise sauce, bacon cheeseburgers." So: no sugars or food made from flour. Atkins even banned fruit juices, and only accepted a minimum of vegetables, although the vegetables became more and more negotiable the longer the diet continued.

Atkins was certainly not the first to become rich by promoting a high-fat diet that limited carbohydrates. But he made it so popular that the American Medical Association considered it a potential threat to our health. The AMA attacked the Atkins diet as a "bizarre diet" that advertised "an unlimited intake of saturated fats and cholesterol-rich foods." Atkins also had to defend his diet in sessions of the American Congress.

Polarization about cause of overweight

Thirty years later, America has become eerily polarized in terms of body weight. On the one hand, everyone is assured with almost religious certainty, from the heart clinic to the general practitioner and we have come to believe with almost religious certainty that excess weight is caused by excessive consumption of fat and that when we reduce eat, lose weight and live longer.

On the other hand, we have the never-ending message from Atkins and decades of best-seller diet books, including "The Zone,"

"Sugar Busters" and "Protein Power" to name just a few. All 'plugs' some variation from what scholars call the alternative hypothesis: it's not the fat that makes us fat, but it's the carbohydrates. If we eat less carbohydrate, we will lose weight and live longer.

The revolutionary of this alternative hypothesis is that it identifies precisely those refined carbohydrates as the cause of overweight, which form the basis of the 'Disc of Five' pasta, rice, and bread. We have always been told that they form the basis of a healthy, low-fat diet. And also the sugar or corn syrup in the lemonades, fruit juices and sports drinks, which we have come to eat in large quantities, for the simple reason that they are fat-free and therefore look good to health.

The less-fat-is-healthy dogma depicts reality as we have come to understand it. And the government has allocated hundreds of millions of dollars to prove its value. In the meantime, the message to eat low-carbohydrates has been referred to the realm of the unscientific fantasy.

More attention for low carb among scientists

However, during the last five years there has been a subtle shift in the scientific consensus. It has long been such that even considering the possibility of the alternative hypothesis, let alone examining it, was equivalent to quackery or complicity with it.

A small but growing group of established scientists are now starting to take seriously into consideration what the low-carb diet researchers have long been proclaiming. Walter Willett, president of the nutrient department at Harvard School of Public Health, is probably the most outspoken advocate of testing this heretical theory. Willet is the mouthpiece of the longest-running, most comprehensive diet and health studies ever conducted, costing more than $100 million and collected data from nearly 300,000 people.

This data, Willett says, clearly contradicts the less-fat-is-healthy message "as well as the idea that all fat is bad for you; the exclusive focus on the adverse effects of fat may have contributed to the obesity epidemic."

These researchers emphasize that there is sufficient reason to believe that the less-fat-is-healthy theory has not stood the test of time. In particular, we are in the midst of an obesity epidemic that began in the early 1980s and coincided with the emergence of the low-fat dogma. (Type II diabetes, the most widespread form of this disease, also increased significantly during this period).

Low fat hopelessly failed

They say that low-fat diets have proven themselves as hopeless failures in clinical trials and in real life. In addition, the percentage of fat in the American diet has been falling for more than two decades. Our cholesterol levels have fallen and we have started smoking less, and the incidence of heart disease has not fallen as we should have expected.

The science behind the alternative hypothesis is called Endocrinology 101, as done by David Ludwig, a researcher at Harvard Medical School, who runs the children's clinic specializing in obesity at Children's Hospital in Boston, and his own version of prescribes a low-carbohydrate diet to his patients.

Endocrinology 101 requires knowledge of how carbohydrates affect insulin and blood sugars and, in turn, fat metabolism and appetite. This is the basis of endocrinology: the study of hormones (such as insulin), says Ludwig. And it is still regarded as radical because the knowledge of the low-fat diet in the 60s came from researchers who were almost exclusively concerned with the effect of fat or cholesterol and heart disease.

Endocrinology 101 was still underdeveloped and was therefore ignored. Now that this science is making progress, it must fight anti-fat prejudices for a quarter of a century.

The alternative hypothesis comes with a result that is worth considering, because it is a 'stunner', and that may be a stumbling block to its acceptance.

If the alternative hypothesis is correct still a big "if" it strongly suggests that the ongoing epidemic of obesity in America and elsewhere, not, as we are constantly told, is simply a consequence of a collective lack of willpower and failure to do physical exercises.

However, it came about, as Atkins claimed all the time (along with Barry Sears, author of "The Zone"), because the government health experts with the best intentions advised us to consume precisely those foods that make us fat, and which we followed. We ate more extra fat-free carbohydrates, which in turn first made us hungry and then heavier.

Simply put, if the alternative hypothesis is correct, then the low-fat diet is not necessarily a healthy diet. In practice, such a diet can only be rich in carbohydrates, which can lead to obesity, perhaps even to heart disease.

Scientific research not easy

Scientists are still bickering about fat, despite a century of research, because the regulation of appetite and weight in the human body appears to be almost incomprehensibly complex and the experimental tools we have to study it are still remarkably inadequate. This combination puts researchers in an unpleasant position. Examine the entire physiological system, which involves feeding real food to real human test subjects for months or years in succession, which is too expensive to perform, ethically unjustifiable (if you want to measure the degree of influence of foods that may cause heart disease) and practically impossible to implement in any scientifically controlled manner.

But if researchers want to carry out a less expensive and more controllable study, this results in the study of experimental situations, which are so much simplified that their results may no longer have anything to do with reality.

This, in turn, leads to a research literature that is so extensive that one can always find some published research to support any theory. The result is a struggling community "shattered, with a rigid opinion and in many cases averse to any compromise," says Kurt Isselbacher, former president of the Food and Nutrition Board of the National Academy of Science. In it researchers seem to be quickly convinced that their preconceived ideas are correct. And they are completely uninterested in investigating any hypothesis other than their own.

Incidentally, the number of misconceptions that are spread over the most basic research is shocking.

Researchers can accurately scientifically describe the limitations of their own experiments, and then proclaim something as the absolute truth because they have read it in a magazine. The classic example is the assertion that is repeatedly heard that 95 percent of all dieters never lose weight, and that 95 percent of those who do, have lost what they have lost.

This is rightly assigned to psychiatrist Albert Stunkard of the University of Pennsylvania, but the statement that this statement is based on 100 patients from Stunkard's obesity clinic during the Eisenhower government (1945-1949) is not included.

It can be said with reservation that one of the few reasonably reliable facts about the obesity epidemic is that it started around the early 1980s. According to what Katherine Flegal said, an epidemiologist at the National Center for Health Statistics, the percentage of Americans with obesity in the 60s and 70s remained relatively constant at 13 to 14 percent and then shot in the 80s by 8 percent up. By the end of that decade, nearly 1 in 4 Americans were obese.

That sharp rise, which prevailed in all layers of the American population and continued uncontrolled during the 90s, is the special feature of the epidemic. Any theory that wants to explain obesity in America will have to account for it. In the meantime, the number of overweight children has almost tripled. And for the first time, doctors started diagnosing Diabetes Type II in growing children. Type II Diabetes is often accompanied by obesity. It used to be called early adult diabetes and now, for explainable reasons, no longer.

Increase in obesity. How could this happen?

The orthodox and generally accepted explanation is that we live in what Kelly Brownell, a Yale psychologist, once called a "toxic food environment" of cheap, fatty food, large portions, penetrating food advertising and sedentary life. According to this theory, we live by the Pavlov-like grace of the food industry, which spends nearly $10 billion a year on advertising unhealthy junk food and fast food.

And because these foods, especially fast foods, are so full of fat, they are both irresistible and extraordinarily fat.

According to this theory, our modern society has also successfully banished the physical exertion from our daily lives. We no longer train and no more stairs, nor do our children cycle to school or play outside, because they prefer to play video games and watch TV.

And because some of us are condemned to become heavier, while others are not, this explanation also has a genetic component the thrift gene. It implies that storing extra calories as fat was an evolutionary benefit for our Paleolithic ancestors, who had to survive frequent famines. So we have inherited these "frugal" genes, despite their danger in today's toxic living environment.

This theory sounds plausible and responds to our Puritan prejudice that fat, fast food and television are extremely harmful to humanity. But there are 2 traps.

First of all, to believe this story, one must accept that the abundant negative reinforcement that accompanies obesity both socially and physically is easily overcome by the constant bombardment of food advertisements and the appeal of a vastly affordable meal.

Secondly, as Flegal points out, there is little information to prove anything of it. At least none of it explains what has changed so remarkably to start the epidemic. Fast food consumption, for example, grew steadily during the 1970s and 1980s, but it did not take a sudden flight, such as obesity.

Regarding training and physical exertion, there is no reliable information from before the mid-80s, according to William Dietz, who heads the nutrition and physical activity department at the Centers for Disease Control; the data from the 90s show the increase in the obesity ratio, while physical activity remained unchanged. This suggests that the two have little agreement.

Dietz also acknowledges that a culture of physical exertion began in the United States in the 1970s the "move-in-your-leisure-mania," such as Robert Levy, director of the National Heart, Lung and Blood Institute, it described in 1981 and continues to date.

As for the 'frugality gene', it offers the kind of evolutionary ratio for human behavior that scientists find reassuring, but that simply cannot be tested. In other words, if we were now in the midst of an anorexia epidemic, the experts would be discussing the equally immeasurable "waste of gene" theory, which proclaims the evolutionary benefits of easy weight loss. An obese homo erectus they would say would have been an easy target for predators.

It is also irrefutable, claim students of Endocrinology 101 that humanity has never evolved to eat a diet rich in starch and sugar.

Low fat only 25 years old

"Cereal products and concentrated sugars were not present in human food until the invention of agriculture," says Ludwig, "which happened only 10,000 years ago."

This is frequently discussed in the anthropology texts, but is absent in the obesity literature, with the obvious exception of the 'Low-Carbohydrate' diet books.

What is overlooked in the current contrast is that the low-fat dogma itself is only about 25 years old. Till the late 70s, the accepted wisdom was that fat and proteins protect against over reacting, because they saturate you and that carbohydrates make you fat.

In "The Physiology of Taste", for example a treatise from 1825 considered to be one of the most famous books ever written about food - French gastronome Jean Anthelme Brillat-Savarin says he could easily identify the causes of obesity, after 30 years of listening to one "set person" after another, the joys of bread, rice and (by a special person) potatoes.

Brillat-Savarin described the roots of obesity as the natural predisposition, combined with the "floral and muddy substances that make them the main ingredient of daily nutrition." He added that the effect of this soggy fare, e.g., "potatoes, grain or any kind of flour" became visible as soon as sugar was supplemented to the diet.

Supported by the vague observation that Italians tend to corpulence because they eat so much pasta. This observation was even documented by Ancel Keys, a doctor from the University of Minnesota, who noted that fats "are firmly on the stomach." By this, he meant that they are being digested slowly and therefore give a satisfying feeling and that Italians were among the heaviest populations that he had studied.

According to Keys, the Neapolitans, for example, only ate a small amount of lean meat once or twice a week, but did eat bread and pasta every day for lunch and dinner. "There was no demonstrable evidence of malnutrition," he wrote, "but the working-class women were fat."

In the 70s there were still articles in the newspapers, which described a high degree of obesity in Africa and the Caribbean, where the diet consisted almost exclusively of carbohydrates. The general opinion, a former director of the Food Department of the United Nations, wrote, was that the ideal diet one that prevented obesity, 'snacking' and abundant sugar consumption was one with 'enough eggs, beef, mutton, chicken, butter and well-cooked vegetables. "This was identical to the prescription Brillat-Savarin stated in 1825.

Influence of politics on low fat

It was notably Ancel Keys, who introduced the less-fat-is-healthy dogma in the 1950s, with his theory that dietary fats increase cholesterol levels and cause heart disease. Over the next two decades, the scientific evidence that this theory was valid remained stubbornly ambiguous.

The matter was ultimately not settled by discoveries, but by politics. It started in January 1977, when a Senate committee led by George McGovern published its "Dietary Prescriptions for the United States" with the advice that Americans drastically reduce their fat intake to an epidemic of "deadly diseases" that plagued the country to stop.

The pinnacle came at the end of 1984 when the National Institutes of Health officially advised that all Americans over the age of 2 should eat less fat. By then, bold had become "the fat killer" to speak in the memorable words of the Center for Science in the Public Interest. And the historic American breakfast of eggs and bacon was well on its way to becoming a bowl of corn flakes with skimmed milk, with a glass of orange juice and toast (without butter) a dubious feast of sophisticated carbohydrates.

In the interceding years, the NIH spent several hundred million dollars trying to prove a connection between eating fat and getting heart disease and, contrary to what we think, they failed. Five major studies revealed no connection whatsoever. However, a sixth, which cost over $100 million, concluded that reducing cholesterol through medication could prevent heart disease. Then the NIH administrators jumped in at the deep end.

Basic Rifkind, who checked the relevant investigations for the NIH, described their logic as follows: they had not succeeded after having spent large sums of money on it, to prove that eating less fat offered any health benefit. But if a cholesterol-lowering drug could stop heart disease, then a low-fat, cholesterol-lowering diet should produce the same result. "The world is simply not perfect," "The data that give a definitive answer is not available, so we must do our best with what is available."

Emerging resistance to low fat

Some of the greatest scientists disagreed with this low-fat logic, claiming that a solid science was incompatible with such a leap in the dark, but they were expertly ignored. Pete Ahrens, whose Rockefeller University lab had done the original research on cholesterol metabolism, explained to McGovern's committee that everyone else responds to a low-fat diet. It was not a question of who might or could not be harmed by it, he said, but "a guess." Phil Handler, when president of the National Academy of Sciences, declared the same in Congress in 1980.

Influence of the food industry on low fat

Nevertheless, now that the NIH had declared itself in favor of the low-fat doctrine, the food industry took over. She quickly started producing thousands of low-fat products to meet the new recommendations. Fat was removed from food such as cookies, chips, and yogurt. The problem was that something else had to replace it, which was tasty and appealing, which meant some form of sugar, often fructose-rich corn syrup.

In the meantime, an entire industry has been established for the manufacture of fat replacements, of which Procter & Gamble's... olestra was the first. And because these low-fat meats, cheeses, snacks, and cookies had to compete with a few hundred thousand other food products sold in America, the industry invested substantial advertising funds in reinforcing the less-fat-is-healthy message.

A great help in this, what Walter Willett calls the "huge amounts" of dietitians, health organizations, consumer groups and even cookbook writers, all well-meaning healthy food missionaries.

Low fat story too simple

Few experts still deny that the low-fat message is presented too simply. At the very least, it very effectively ignores the fact that unsaturated fats, such as olive oil, are relatively healthy for you: they tend to raise good cholesterol (HDL) and lower bad cholesterol (LDL), at least in proportion to its effect of carbohydrates. While a higher LDL level increases the risk of heart disease, it is slowed by a higher HDL level.

What that means is that even saturated fats alias the 'bad' fats are not as harmful as we think. Indeed, they increase your cholesterol level, but at the same time, they will raise the 'good' cholesterol level. In other words, it doesn't matter. As Willet explained, you will achieve little or no health improvement by leaving milk, butter, and cheese to eat bagels instead.

But it gets even crazier. Nutrients that were considered more or less deadly under the low-fat dogma appear to be relatively benign when you look at their current fat content. More than 2/3 of the fat in a Porterhouse Steak, for example, will improve your cholesterol profile (at least in proportion to the baked potato that is next to it); the remainder of the LDL the bad stuff will indeed increase, but it will also raise your HDL. The same applies to pork fat. If you do the numerical work, you come to the surrealistic conclusion that you can eat pork fat from the package in this way, while considerably reducing your chance of heart disease.

The crucial instance of how the low-fat recommendations have been simplified is the impact (potentially life-threatening incidentally) of low-fat diets on triglycerides, which are the binding molecules of fat. By the end of the 1960s, scientists had proven that high triglyceride levels were at least as common in patients with heart disease as high LDL cholesterol levels. And that eating low-fat, carbohydrate-rich foods would increase their triglyceride levels, lower their HDL levels, and accentuate what Gerry Reaven, an endocrinologist at Stanford University, calls Syndrome X. This is a group of conditions that can lead to heart disease and Type 2 diabetes.

Eating low fat and high carb causes a health problem

It took Reaven a year to convince his environment that Syndrome X was a legitimate health problem. "Sometimes we wish it would just disappear because nobody knows what to do with it," said Robert Silverman, and NIH researcher, at an NIH conference in 1987. "Great protein levels can be critical for the kidneys. High-fat content is bad for the heart. Now Reaven tells us not to use large amounts of carbohydrate. We have to eat something. "

Certainly, everyone involved in the composition of the various dietary recommendations simply wanted Americans to eat less junk food. However, you want to define it, and to eat more as is done in Berkeley, California. But we didn't go along with it. Instead, we ate more starches and processed carbohydrates, because these, calorie by calorie, are the cheapest foods that the food industry can produce. And they can be sold with the most profit. It is also what we love to eat. The person below the age of

50 who do not prefer a cookie or sweetened yogurt over a broccoli sprout, is very rare.

The food industry sees its chance as clean

"All researchers would do well to become aware of the law of unintended consequences," said Alan Stone, who was the director of the McGovern Senate Committee. Stone told me he already suspected how the food industry would react to the new dietary advice when the hearings were first held.

An economist took him aside, he said, and gave him a lesson in marketing healthy eating: "He said: create a new market with brand-new food produced, give it a brand new, chic name, put a big advertising budget behind it, then you have the market all to yourself, and you can force your competitors to catch up. You can't do that with fruit and vegetables. It is harder to make a difference between an apple and an apple. "

Nutritionists also played a role because they tried to get science to assume that carbohydrates are the ideal food. That fat counts nine calories per gram, compared to four for carbohydrates and proteins. Was known for almost a century. It was generally considered irrelevant for research into the causes of obesity. So now the safe proposition of the low-fat recommendations became: reduce the main source of dietary calories, and you will lose weight.

In 1982, JP Flatt, a biochemist at the University of Massachusetts, published his research, in which he demonstrated that in a normal diet it is very rare for the human body to transform carbohydrates into body fat. This was then distorted by the media and a large number of scientists, in the sense that eating carbohydrates, even in excessive amounts, cannot make them fat which is not the case, Flatt says.

But the misunderstanding began to lead a powerful life of its own because it coincided with the view that fat leads to obesity and that carbohydrates are harmless.

As a result, according to USDA agricultural economist Judith Putnam, the most important development in the American diet since the end of the 1970s has been a reduction in the percentage of fat calories and a "very extended consumption of carbohydrates." To be precise, seasonal grain consumption has risen by almost 30 kilos per person and calorie-rich sweeteners (mainly fructose-rich corn syrup) by 15 kilos.

At the same time, we suddenly started to consume more calories: now up to 400 more a day since the government started recommending low-fat diets.

If these trends are correct, the fat epidemic can be explained by Americans eating more calories than ever before unnecessary calories, after all, make us gain weight and in particular, more carbohydrates.

The question is, why?

The answer given by Endocrinology 101 is that we are simply hungrier than in the 1970s. And the reason for that is physiological, rather than psychological. In this case, the saturation factor ignored in the hunt for fat, and its effect on cholesterol is how carbohydrates affect blood sugar and insulin.

These were already the designated culprits, so Atkins and the low-carb diet doctors jumped up early.

The primary task of insulin

After you have eaten carbohydrates, they are broken down into sugar molecules and transported to the bloodstream. The pancreas then secretes insulin, which brings blood sugar into the muscles and liver as fuel for the coming hours. For this reason, carbohydrates have a significant effect on insulin and not fat. And since a lack of insulin causes childhood diabetes, doctors believe since the 1920s that the only problem you can have with insulin is that you are not tired of it.

But insulin also regulates fat metabolism. We cannot store body fat without insulin. Imagine your insulin as a switch. If it is on, those few hours after a meal, you burn carbohydrates as energy, and you store excess calories as fat. If it is off after the insulin has been used up, you burn fat as fuel, so if the insulin level is low, you are going to burn your fat, but not if it is high.

And now it is necessarily complicated. The thicker you are, the more insulin your pancreas produces per meal, and the more likely it is that you will develop a so-called "insulin resistance," which is the underlying cause of Syndrome X.

Your cells become indifferent to the action of the insulin, and therefore, you need larger quantities to regulate your blood sugar. Thus, as you gain weight, insulin makes it easier to store fat and harder to lose. But insulin resistance, in turn, may make it harder to store fat your weight will stay the way it should be. But now the insulin resistance would probably stimulate your pancreas to produce even more insulin, so the potential start of a vicious circle.

What comes first obesity, increased insulin levels, called 'hyperinsulinism,' or insulin resistance is a matter of chicken and egg, which has not been resolved. An endocrinologist described this as "a problem whose solution deserves the Nobel prize."

Effect of insulin on feeling hungry

Insulin also greatly influences hunger for what purpose that happens is another point of contention. On the one hand, insulin can diffusely cause hunger because it lowers your blood sugar level. But how low do you need to get blood sugar before the hunger strikes? That is still unresolved. In the meantime, insulin operates in the brain to suppress hunger.

The method, as explained to me by Michael Schwartz, an endocrinologist at the University of Washington, is that the ability of insulin to suppress appetite normally counteracts its ability to generate body fat. In other words, as you gain weight, your body produces more insulin with every meal, which in turn would suppress your appetite; you would eat less and lose weight.

Schwartz, though, can imagine a simple mechanism that brings this "homeostatic" system out of balance: if your brain loses its sensitivity to insulin, just like your fat and muscles do if they are flooded with it.

Now the higher insulin production associated with getting fatter is no longer compensated by inhibiting your appetite because your brain no longer records the increase in insulin levels.

The result is a physiological condition in which obesity is a logical consequence and one in which the carbohydrate-insulin ratio can play a major role. Schwartz says he believes this is indeed happening, but science is not yet far enough advanced to prove it. "It's just a hypothesis," he says, "It needs to be investigated further."

David Ludwig, endocrinologist at Harvard, says it is the direct effect of insulin on blood sugar that it does. He writes that when diabetics get much insulin, their blood sugar plummets and they get wildly hungry. They arrive because they eat more, and insulin also promotes fat production.

The same happens with laboratory animals. This, he says, is actually what happens when we eat carbohydrates especially sugar and starches such as potatoes and rice, or something made from flour, such as a slice of white bread. These are identified in the jargon as high-glycemic-index carbohydrates, which mean that the blood rapidly absorbs them.

Vicious circle

The result is a blood sugar peak and an influx of insulin within minutes. The influx of insulin lowers your blood sugar, and a few hours later, your blood sugar is lower than it was before you ate. As Ludwig explains, your body thinks the fuel has run out, but the insulin is still high enough to prevent you from burning your fat. The result is hunger and a desire for more carbohydrates. It is another vicious circle and another situation that is ripe for obesity.

The glycemic index concept and the idea that starches can be absorbed into the bloodstream even faster than sugar originated in the late 70s, but again did not influence public health recommendations, due to the controversies present.

Imagine: if you accepted the glycemic index concept, you also had to accept that once the starches, which were supposed to be eaten 6 to 11 times a day, were swallowed; they could not be distinguished physiologically from sugar. This made them considerably less healthy. Rather than accepting this possibility, the politicians let sugar and corn syrup escape from the defamation that fats had. After all, they are fat-free.

Sugar and corn syrup in lemonades, juices and copious meals and sports drinks now provide more than 10 percent of our total calorie intake.

In the 1980s, for example, Coca-Cola liter bottles were introduced, chock-full of sugar but 100 percent fat-free. As far as insulin and blood sugars are concerned, these soft drinks and fruit juices scientists call them "wet carbohydrates" may be the worst of all. (Light drinks cover less than a quarter of the soft drinks market).

The purpose of the glycemic index is that the longer carbohydrates take to be digested, the less the influence on blood sugar and insulin, and the healthier the food. The foods at the top of the glycemic index are simple sugars, starches, and anything produced from flour.

Green vegetables, beans, and grains cause a much slower rise in blood sugar because they contain fiber, an indigestible carbohydrate. This makes the digestion slower and lowers the glycemic index. Protein and fat have the same effect, meaning that eating fat can be healthy, an idea that is still unacceptable. And the glycemic index concept means that the primary cause of

Syndrome X, heart disease, Type 2 diabetes, and obesity is the long-term damage caused by repeated spikes of insulin that result from consuming starches and refined carbohydrates. This suggests a more or less unequivocal theory for all these chronic diseases, but not one that easily falls within the low-fat doctrine.

In his overweight youth clinic, Ludwig has been prescribing low-glycemic index diets for children and growing youth for five years. He does not suggest the Atkins diet because he claims to believe that such a low carbohydrate approach is unnecessarily restrictive; instead, he advises his patients to replace the refined carbohydrates and starches with fruit and vegetables.

This becomes a low-glycemic-index diet that corresponds to dietary logic, albeit in a more fat-rich way.

His clinic presently has a nine-month waiting list. Only recently has Ludwig succeeded in convincing the NIH that such diets are worth studying. His first three proposals were rejected, which may explain why most of the relevant research was done in Canada and Australia.

In April, however, Ludwig accepted $1.2 million from the NIH to test his low-glycemic-index diet against a low-fat-low-calorie regime. That may help to solve some of the controversies over the role of insulin in obesity, although the dreaded Dr. Atkins may be quicker to finish.

Dr. Atkins: eat few carbohydrates

71-year-old Atkins, a Ph.D. at Cornell medical school, says he first tried a very low-carb diet in 1963 after reading about it in the Journal of the American Medical Association. He lost weight effortlessly, saw the 'light' and turned a starting cardiological practice in Manhattan into a thriving obesity clinic.

He then chased the entire medical world against him, advising his readers to eat just as much fat and protein as they wanted, as long as they ate little or no carbs. They would lose weight, he said, because both kept their insulin levels low; they would not be hungry, and they would experience less resistance when burning their fat.

Atkins also indicated that starches and sugar were harmful in any case because they increase triglyceride levels. This is a greater risk of heart disease than cholesterol.

Atkins' diet is both the ultimate manifestation of the alternative hypothesis and the arena in which the fat-versus-carbohydrate controversy is likely to be fought in the coming years. After claiming for 30 years that Atkins was a charlatan, overweight experts now find it difficult to ignore the frequent and anecdotal evidence that his diet does exactly what he claimed.

Take Albert Stunkard, for example. He has been trying to treat obesity for half a century, but he told me that the penny fell on Atkins and perhaps on obesity only recently, when he discovered that the head radiologist at his hospital had lost 60 pounds. Thanks to the Atkins diet. "Well, it seems that all the young guys in the hospital are following it," he said, "so we decided to do a study."

When asked Stunkard if he or one of his colleagues had considered testing Atkins' diet thirty years ago, he said that this was not the case because they thought Atkins was "a creep" who was only out for To earn money. "This repelled people, and that is why nobody took him seriously enough to do what we are finally doing."

By the way, when the American Medical Association expressed its devastating criticism of Atkins' diet in March '73, they acknowledged that the diet would probably work, but showed no interest in the why. During the 1960s, this had been the subject of thorough research, with the conclusion that diets such as those of Atkins were disguised low-calorie diets. When you exclude pasta, bread, and potatoes, it becomes difficult to eat enough meat, vegetables, and cheese to replace those calories.

However, that raises the question of why such a low-calorie diet would also suppress hunger, which according to Atkins was the characteristic of his diet. One probability was Endocrinology 101: that fat and proteins saturate you and that you remain saturated due to a lack of carbohydrates and the subsequent fluctuation in blood sugar and insulin.

The other possibility came from the fact that Atkins' diet is' ketogenic.' This means that the insulin level drops so low that you get into a state of ketosis, which also happens during fasting and famine. Your muscles and fibers burn body fat for energy, as your brain does in the form of fat molecules called ketones that are produced by the liver. Atkins saw ketosis as the logical way to initiate weight loss.

He used to say that ketosis gave so much energy that it was even better than sex, for which he was often laughed at.

An inevitable criticism of Atkins' diet was that ketosis would be dangerous and should be avoided at all costs.

When interviewed ketosis experts, they all agreed with Atkins and suggested that the medical world and the media regard ketosis as ketoacidosis, a variant of ketosis that occurs in untreated diabetics and can be fatal.

"Doctors are afraid of ketosis," says Richard Veech, an NIH researcher who studied medicine at Harvard and then obtained a Ph.D. at Oxford University with Nobel Prize winner Hans Krebs. "They are always worried about diabetic ketoacidosis. But ketosis is a normal physiological condition. Ketosis is the normal state of humanity. It is not natural to have a McDonald and a takeaway restaurant on every street corner. Normál is to suffer worse.

Simply put, ketosis is the answer of evolution to the frugality gene. We may have evolved so that we can store fat for times of food scarcity, Veech says, but we've also evolved ketosis to live efficiently from that fat if needed. Instead of being poison, as the press often portrays it, fat makes the body work more efficiently and provides a reserve of fuel for the brain. Veech calls ketones "panacea" and has shown that both the heart and brain function 25 percent more efficiently on ketones than on blood sugar.

that For nearly 30 years, Atkins maintained that his diet worked and was safe, and apparently tens of millions of Americans tried it out, while nutritionists, doctors, official health experts, and anyone who had anything to do with heart disease, vowed to kill would be, but showed little or no urge to find out who was right now.

During that period, only two groups of American researchers tested the diet; at least only two groups published their results.

In the early 1970s, JP Flatt and Harvard's George Blackburn pioneered "protein-sparing modified fast" (translator's note: these are replacement meals as an alternative to total fasting.

The diet was "lean meat, fish and poultry" supplemented with vitamins and minerals. "People loved it," Blackburn remembers. "Fantastic weight loss. The people were not to be missed". Blackburn successfully treated hundreds of obese patients in the next 10 years and published a series of articles that were ignored.

When New Englanders started using appetite-suppressing drugs in the mid-1980s, he stopped. He then applied to the NIH for a grant to do a clinical test with popular diets, but it was rejected.

The second study, published in September 1980, was conducted at the George Washington University Medical Center. Two dozen obese volunteers agreed to follow Atkins' diet for eight weeks and lost an average of 8 pounds per person, with no obvious drawbacks, although their LDL cholesterol did rise.

The researchers, supervised by John LaRosa, now president of the State University of New York Downstate Medical Center in Brooklyn, resolved that the weight loss of 8 pounds in eight weeks would probably have happened to any diet by "trying out the novelty of something under experimental conditions" and didn't spend any further attention to it.

Finally an investigation into the Atkins diet

Now researchers have finally decided that the Atkins diet and other low-carbohydrate diets should be investigated, and are now doing so against traditional low-calorie and low-fat diets, as recommended by the American Heart Association.

To explain their motivation, they always tell one of two stories: Some, like Stunkard, told me that someone they knew a patient, a friend, another doctor had lost considerable weight due to the Atkins diet and, despite all the prejudices it contrary, had not recovered.

Others say that they were frustrated by their inability to help obese patients, immersed themselves in low-carbohydrate diets and found that Endocrinology 101 appealed to them. "As a doctor, I was taught to honing all diets such as Atkins," says Linda Stern, an internist at the Philadelphia Veterans Administration Hospital, "but I started the diet myself. It went fantastic. And I thought that maybe this was something I could offer my patients".

The NIH has funded none of these studies, and none have already been published. But the results were announced at conferences by researchers at the Schneider Children's Hospital on Long Island, Duke University and the University of Cincinnati, and by Stern's group at the Philadelphia VA Hospital.

And then there's the research that Stunkard mentioned, led by Gary Foster at the University of Pennsylvania, Sam Klein, director of the Center for Human Nutrition at Washington University in St. Louis, and Jim Hill, who is the University of Colorado Center for Human Nutrition in Denver leads.

Dr. Atkins diet across the board better than a low-fat diet

The results of all five studies are remarkably consistent. Subjects are taking some form of the Atkins diet either obese adolescents who followed the diet for 12 weeks at Schneider, or obese adults with an average weight of 140 kg, who did the diet for six months, such as the Philadelphia VA twice as many as the subjects who did the low-fat and low-calorie diets.

In all five studies, cholesterol levels improved in the same way for both diets, but the triglyceride level was considerably lower with the Atkins diet. Although the researchers hesitate to agree, it would suggest that the risk of heart disease can be reduced if fat is added back to the food and the carbohydrates removed. "I think once this is acknowledged," says Stunkard, "it will turn thinking about obesity and metabolism upside down."

This should all be arranged as quickly as possible, with which we may perhaps receive a few long-awaited answers to questions such as: why we get fat and whether it is indeed predisposed by social circumstances or by our food choice.

For the first time, the NIH is funding comparative studies of popular diets. For example, Foster, Klein, and Hill have now received more than $2.5 million from the NIH to do a 5-year study of the Atkins diet with 360 obese people. At Harvard, Willett, Blackburn and Penelope Green have also received money to do a comparative study, albeit from Atkins' nonprofit foundation.

Should these clinical trials also prove beneficial to Atkins and his high-fat, low-carbohydrate diet, the public health authorities have a problem.

When they spoke in good faith before the low-fat dogma 25 years ago, they left little room for opposite evidence or a change of opinion, if such a change were necessary to keep up with science.

In this light, Sam Klein's experience is remarkable. Klein is the future president of the North American Association for the Study of Obesity, suggesting that he is a highly respected member of this organization. And yet he described his recent experience of discussing the Atkins diet during a medical conference as an instructive experience. "I am impressed," he said, "of the unadorned wrath of the academics. Their response is: How dare you present any data about the Atkins diet! ".

ATKINS DIET: ALLOWED FOOD

What can one eat in the Atkins diet? The diet plan

The good news is that the Atkins diet allows for a lot of things that are taboo on most other diets. You can eat or drink fatty sausages, red meat, full-fat dairy products, and certain types of alcohol, for example - but you have to do without other tasty things completely and permanently.

The Atkins shopping list

Not all foods from the following list are allowed at any time of the diet. Whole milk products and fruit are not provided for example in Phase 1, but may still be on the shopping list for the time after entry. In the Atkins diet, you can eat the following foods:

- Meat (various sorts, also red meat)
- sausage
- fish
- Vegetables that grow above the earth, including preferably all kinds of salad or cabbage as well as cucumber, peppers, leeks, spinach, pumpkin or carrots
- Soy products
- eggs
- Coffee or caffeine in the form of black/green tea
- Oils and fats (coconut oil, olive oil, sesame oil, lard, mayonnaise, ...)
- Alcohol (sherry, dry/semi-dry white wine, beer, red wine, sparkling wine, champagne)

- Dairy products (pasture butter, whole milk, cream, buttermilk, various cheeses, yogurt)

Fruits (papaya, avocado, berries, citrus fruits such as orange, lemon or grapefruit, kiwi)

The range of products allowed is therefore not necessarily small, but you must pay attention to the carbohydrate content of your meals in the individual diet phases. And of course, it's not about stuffing as much fat as possible on each diet day.

Forbidden foods in the Atkins diet

The low carb diet is designed to prevent the body from gaining energy from carbohydrates accordingly, the list of prohibited foods in the Atkins diet. Deleted are:

- Bread and other varieties of pastry
- pasta
- Other cereal products (couscous, bulgur, quinoa, etc.)
- rice
- Sugar, also in the form of fruits / dried fruits or natural sweetness (maple syrup, honey, etc.)

So, if you like it sweet, you're at a disadvantage with the Atkins diet, because you want to eliminate all kinds of sweeteners. After all, fruit and thus fructose is allowed from phase 4 of the diet again in moderation. The situation is different with cakes and co. Because these foods should be painted as completely as possible.

Since then the so-called attacks ketosis one: With the dramatic shutdown of carbohydrates at the beginning of the body gets problems to get to enough energy, so he developed a contingency plan and uses fat from the diet directly as an energy source and also builds intercalated fat off for energy. Normally your body would go to the muscles with too few carbs, so energy sources, to gain new energy from the protein of the muscles. Due to the high fat and protein intake from your Meals, the body does not go to your muscles.

KETOSIS: WHAT WAS THAT EXACTLY AGAIN?

Short Digression: The preferred energy of your body is carbohydrates. The carbs are broken down into specific sugar molecules, glucose, and are released into the blood. The blood sugar level rises, and your pancreas produces the so-called memory hormone insulin. It ensures that the energy in the form of sugar is transported into the cells. In particular, your brain relies on carbs. The downside: if your muscle cells and your brain do not consume the energy completely, it will be stored very quickly as an extra cushion in the fat cells.

Here is the ketosis help: By your body's favorite source of energy carbohydrates take away, he must look for an alternative source of energy and what is more obvious than to choose fat? Of that, you provide him on the fat-based diet much available and also has your body own large stores on the stomach, hips, and buttocks. For energy to be produced from fats, the body has developed a contingency plan called ketosis. Your body produces so-called ketone bodies in the liver from the free fatty acids of your fat cells; this is a water-soluble glucose alternative that is well transported in the blood and can cross the blood-brain barrier so that your brain gets the much-needed energy. In ketosis, you draw your energy from fats and not from the body's protein, the muscles. The ketogenic diet, therefore, promises fat loss without muscle loss! By the way: ketone bodies should provide about 25% more energy than glucose and also much more even.

The ketosis begins as soon as your insulin level falls below a certain value. When this value is reached varies from person to person, but there is the possibility of finding out about blood, urine, or breath tests. However, whether you are in ketosis, you also notice physical symptoms such as increased urination, dry mouth, great thirst, less hunger, bad breath, strange taste in the mouth and increased concentration and energy.

Likewise, when ketosis ceases, dry eyes, bad sleep, (hot) hunger, and a sudden, heavy increase in weight are possible signs.

Ketosis is also reached if you do not eat for a long time. Therefore it is also called "hunger metabolism" and seen as an imitation of fasting metabolism. When your body is in ketosis for long periods, keto-adaptation is used: your body has switched its primary source of energy from carbs to fats. While this is not completely the case with the Atkins diet, with a completely ketogenic diet a three-month ketosis phase is being discussed, but your body is still learning to use the fats as an energy source. Later in the Atkins diet, the carbs gradually become smaller in moderation to the extent that will not let you increase again. The ketosis is then stopped again; it is used in the diet so only for losing weight.

HOW IS THE ATKIN'S DIET DIFFERENT FROM THE KETOGENIC DIET?

It can be easy to get confused with these two diet plans because both focus on the consumption of low carbohydrates. However, there are still a few distinctions about each of them.

Ketogenic diets are based on the principles of eating a specific amount or a percentage of the macronutrients in your daily diet. It enables you to eat a lot of fat up to 60%, an adequate amount of protein around 35 %, while only encouraging very low carbohydrate consumption by only 5 %. This helps force the body to ketosis, where it uses "ketones" as an When there are not enough carbohydrates in the body for a prolonged period, the body through the liver enters our fat deposits and begins to convert fats into fatty acids and ketones that it uses as energy. This process helps the body lose a large amount of fat when it is in ketosis.

The Atkins diet also gives a promising result when it comes to losing weight, but it allows you to eat as much fat and protein as you want since you only consume a small number of carbohydrates.

The diet is a product of Dr. Robert Coleman Atkins, an American doctor, and cardiologist, and is a diet that involves starting with ketosis and staying in ketosis until you have lost a considerable amount of weight. This is called the "induction" phase of the diet. After induction, gradually reintroduce carbohydrates, making sure they are still low in carbohydrates and avoid carbohydrates and unwanted processed sugars. And that is one of the main differences between Ketosis and Atkins.

Ketosis is a very effective way to lose weight since it is the metabolism of starvation. Your body stops trying to burn sugars as fuel and begins to burn your fat reserves.

Few differences between them:

- Ketogenic is 60% fat, while Atkins allows unlimited fat consumption
- Ketogenic allows 35% protein while Atkins allows unlimited protein consumption
- Ketogenic allows 5% carbohydrates, while Atkins allows just under 50g of carbohydrates
- Atkins is more comfortable to follow than the ketogenic diet and a short-term weight loss diet, but it also comes with different health risks
- The ketogenic diet is a more precise way of eating to change your metabolism
- The ketogenic diet offers much better long-term health benefits once you get used to implementing it in your life.

Related of "How is the Atkin's diet different from the ketogenic diet?"

The ketogenic diet is VERY specific about the proportion of macronutrients and is in a state of ketosis (hence the name of the diet). While Atkins is not like that, it is a low carb diet with different "carbohydrate allocation phases."

Ketogenic diet Fat / Protein / Carbohydrate: 75% + / 15-20% / 5-10%

Atkins is not so strict with macros. It is more a low carb diet, when you specifically restrict the number of carbohydrates, not necessarily tracking the intake of fats and proteins as much.

Atkins especially modified and new, although it is also about putting your body in a metabolic state in which you burn fat as your main source of fuel.

At the moment Atkins and Keto make a kind of mixture with all the modified versions, keto and Atkins cycling, etc.

Having said that, from memory the key distinction I remember is that, while a ketogenic diet is low in carbohydrates (and that is why I mean at least below 50 g / day, for some even less), modest protein (limited to avoid too much excess protein that can result in gluconeogenesis, resulting in increased blood sugar and insulin, etc.) and high fat content, the Atkins diet is high in fat, high in protein and low in in carbohydrates.

Also, the truly low carbohydrate period in Atkins lasts only the first 2 weeks, after which it begins to add more starchy vegetables to your diet slowly. In a ketogenic diet, you continue to maintain your carbohydrate intake generally low essentially undefined, although, of course, you can cycle from time to time or allow yourself more freedom than at the beginning concerning carbohydrates (which is fine if has been adapted, etc. of course)

Therefore, to clarify, a ketogenic diet keeps you in nutritional ketosis, regardless of your intake of carbohydrates and proteins, but begins as low in carbohydrates, high in fat and moderate in protein.

DIET OF KETONIC VS. ATKINS

The Atkins diet is a low carb diet, but the difference is in the number of proteins and carbohydrates that you can ingest per day.

The Atkins diet is based mainly on proteins, while the ketogenic diet suggests an average protein intake.

Main differences

- Ketogenic suggest about 65% fat, while Atkins allows unlimited fat consumption
- Keto allows up to 40% protein, while Atkins allows unlimited protein consumption
- Ketogenic allows 5% carbohydrates - Atkins allows 50 g of carbohydrates

Atkins is more comfortable to follow than the ketogenic diet, but it also presents different health risks. The keto diet gives much better long-term health benefits.

Phase 1 of Atkins is a ketogenic diet.

The next 3 phases will gradually reintroduce carbohydrates into your diet.

List of healthy foods of carbohydrates and dietary foods

Paleo and ketogenic diets are similar, even Atkins is similar if you look at their principles? Yes, there are slight differences that are important because they achieve very different objectives.

The Atkins diet is based mainly on proteins, that is, eating as much protein as you want and without sugars.

Ketogenic is: eat 25 g or less of carbohydrates per day, adequate amounts of protein per day, usually around 1 g per kg of body weight, and the amount of fat you want.

Simple

Atkins says to eat all the protein you want. Modern ketogenic diets emphasize fats and recommend only moderate amounts of protein.

Atkins is low in carbohydrates, but Keto has less than 25 grams of net carbohydrates and uses a more fat-rich approach.

QUICHE WITH SPINACH, MUSHROOMS & FETA

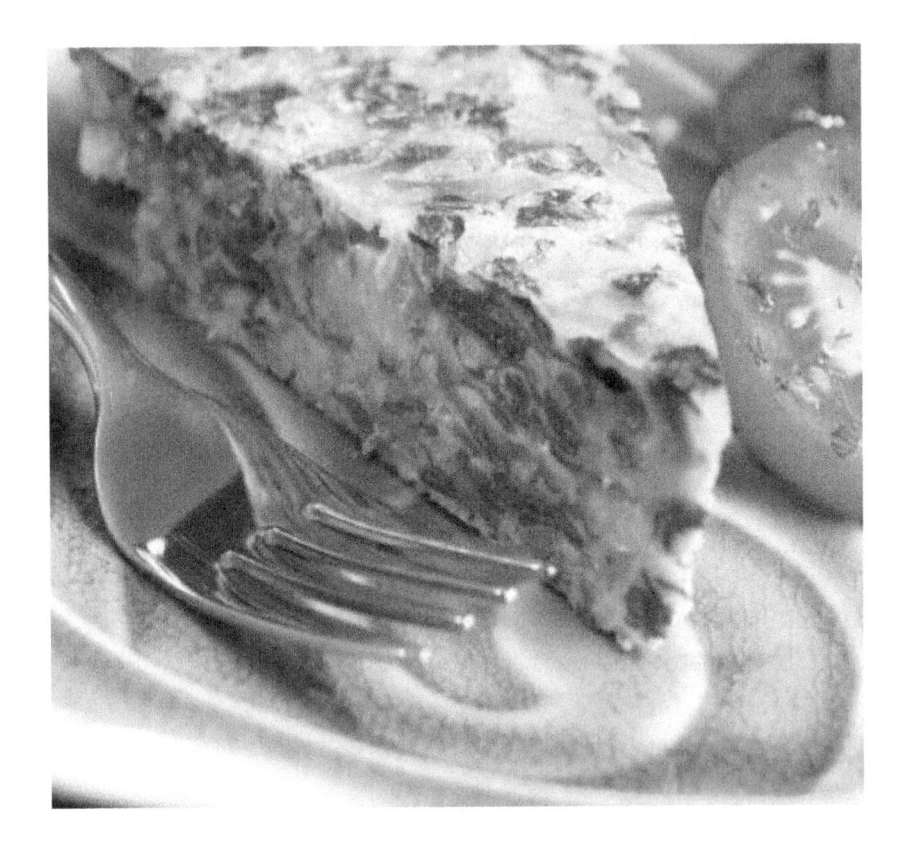

Servings: 4

Preparation time: 20 minutes

Cooking time: 55 minutes

Nutritional Fact: Carbohydrates: 3g

INGREDIENTS

- 150 grams of mushrooms
- 2 cloves of garlic
- 200 grams of spinach
- 3 eggs
- 150 ml unsweetened almond milk
- 50 grams of feta cheese
- 3 tablespoons of Parmesan
- 1 teaspoon salt
- 1 teaspoon of black pepper
- 50 grams of mozzarella

PREPARATION

1. Preheat the oven. Slice the mushrooms and garlic in thin slices. Put them together with salt & pepper in a greased frying pan and sweat for about 5 minutes until soft. Grease a baking dish, first add the spinach to the baking dish and then add the mushrooms and feta cheese. Then add the eggs, milk, and Parmesan together in a bowl. Season something with pepper. Pour the egg mixture into the mold and sprinkle with the grated mozzarella. Bake the quiche for 45 - 55 minutes or until the cheese is golden brown

EGGS BAKED IN AVOCADO

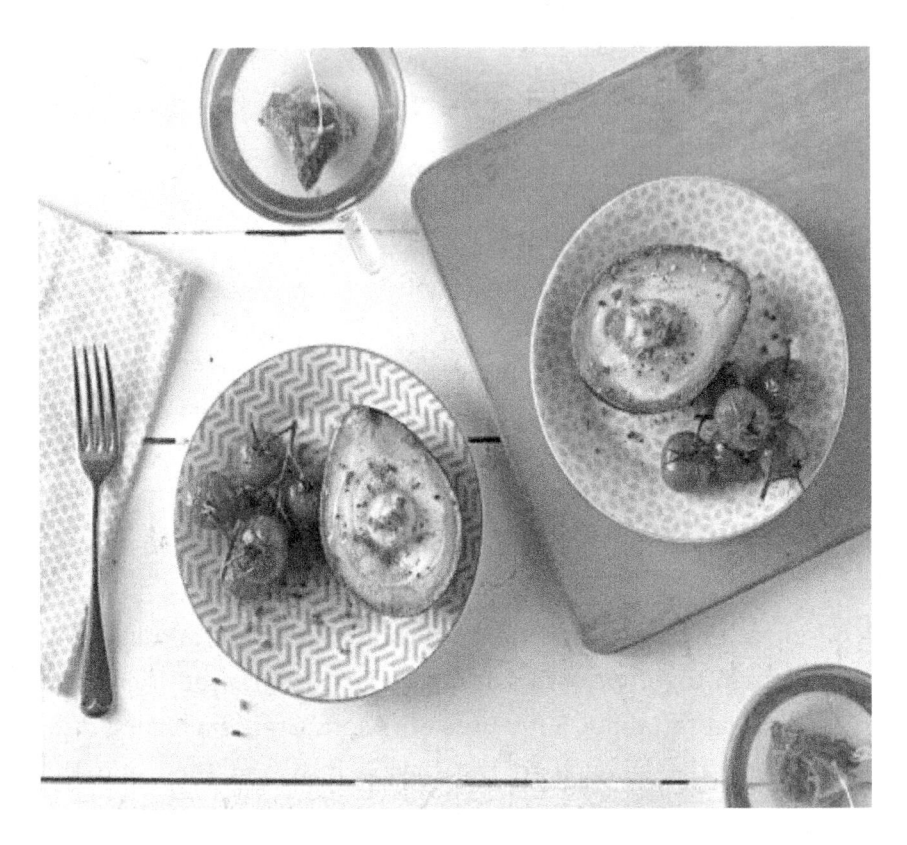

This is a typical low carbohydrate dish. Eggs contain a lot of protein, so they fit wonderfully into your low carbohydrate lifestyle. Not only is it a healthy and delicious dish, but it also looks great!

Servings: 2

Preparation time: 5 minutes

Cooking time: 25 minutes

Nutritional Fact: Carbohydrates: 2g

INGREDIENTS

- 2 eggs
- 1 avocado
- 1 teaspoon salt
- 1 teaspoon of black pepper
- 1 tablespoon of fresh chives

PREPARATION

1. Preheat the oven. Halve the avocado and remove the core. Pick up about two tablespoons of the meat from the middle of the avocado, just enough to make the egg fit right in the middle. Then put them in a small baking dish.
2. Make an egg in each avocado half. Try to put the yolk in the cavity first, and then add the egg whites to fill in the rest.
3. Put in the oven and bake for 15 to 20 minutes. The cooking time depends on the size of the eggs and avocados. Make sure that the protein has enough time to sit down. Remove from the oven and season with salt, pepper, and chives.

CRUNCHY CHOCOLATE COVERED STRAWBERRIES

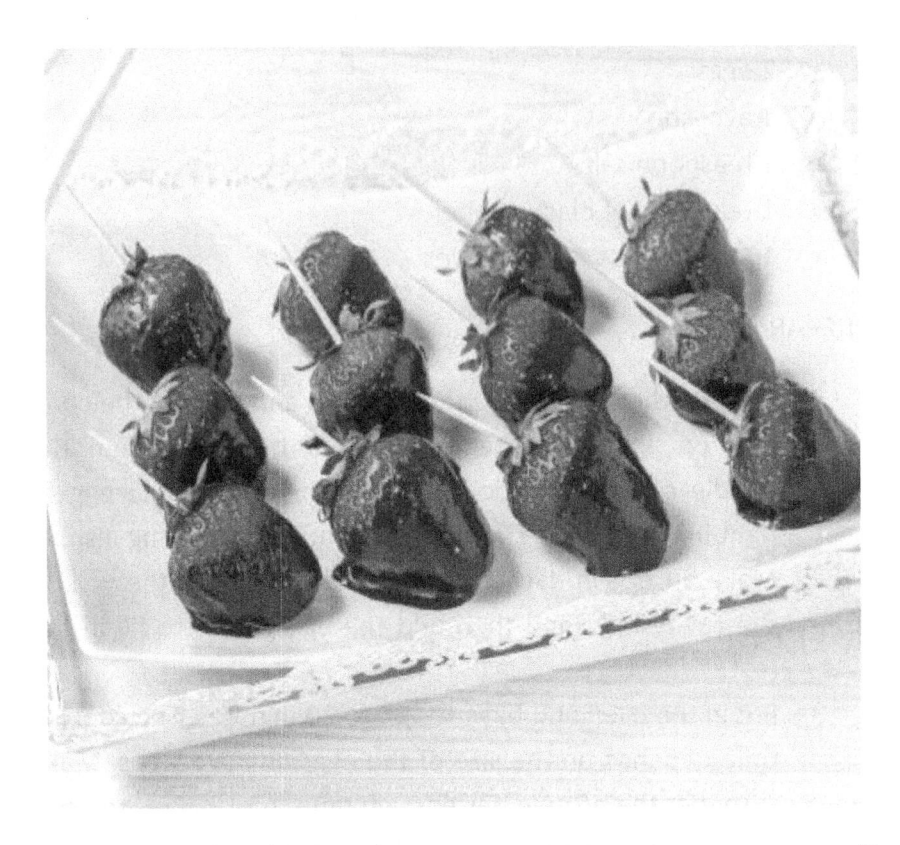

Share this dish with a loved one as a special treat or treat yourself to something good with this simple dessert!

Servings: 2

Preparation time: 10 mins

Cooking time: 10 mins

Nutritional Fact: Carbohydrates: 12g

INGREDIENTS

- 10 fresh strawberries
- 1 Atkins crispy milk chocolate bar

PREPARATION

1. Lay out a baking tray with baking paper. Break the Atkins bar into even pieces and place it in a heat-resistant bowl (take one that fits your pot).
2. Fill a pot 1/3 with water; bring the water to a boil. Once cooked, reduce the heat. Place the bowl over the pot - make sure the bowl does not come into contact with the water. Stir the chocolate with a metal spoon until completely melted and smooth.
3. Dip each strawberry about 2/3 into the melted chocolate, keeping it at the top, then place it on the baking paper. Repeat for all strawberries.
4. Put the strawberries in the fridge to cool.
5. Use the remaining chocolate to decorate your platter.

FISH PIE

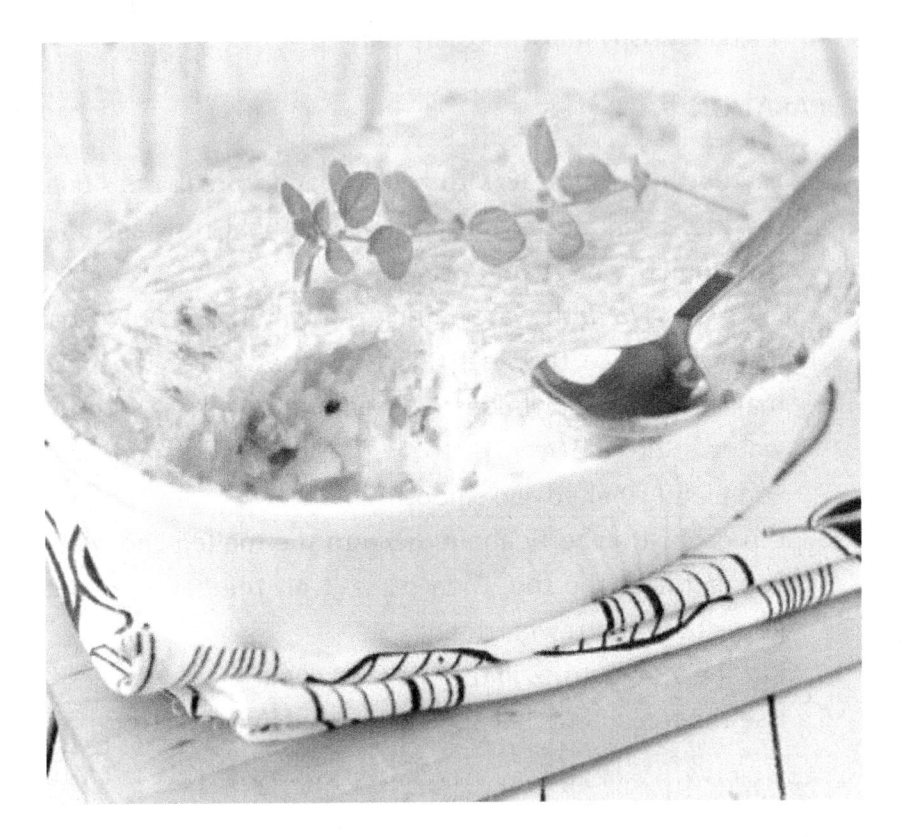

Fancy a delicious fish cake? Try this recipe with some salmon, white fish, tomatoes and spices. A great meal to prepare for a cozy dinner with friends. Healthy and naturally low carb.

Servings: 4

Preparation time: 10 mins

Cooking time: 60 minutes

Nutritional Fact: Carbohydrates: 5g

INGREDIENTS

- 1 tablespoon of olive oil
- 50 grams of white onion
- 2 cloves of garlic
- 400 grams of canned tomatoes
- 1 tablespoon of fresh ginger
- 1 teaspoon of cinnamon powder
- 1 teaspoon salt
- 1 teaspoon of black pepper
- 150 grams of salmon fillet
- 150 grams of white fish fillet
- 2 tablespoons butter
- 100 grams of celery

PREPARATION

1. Preheat the oven to gas level 3 or 175 ° C. Chop the celery and cook for 7 - 10 minutes in salted water. Pass, purée, and mix in the butter. Taste it with salt and pepper. Put the fish in a pot of boiling water, with just enough water to cover it. Cook for 5 minutes. The fish should be dark and easily disintegrate. Drain the fish and put it in a bowl. Put the oil in a pan over medium heat and sweat the onion and garlic for 5 minutes. Stir in the boiled fish, chopped tomatoes, cinnamon, ginger, salt, and pepper. Let it simmer over medium heat to allow the flavors to develop. Put the mass in a small frying pan and cover with the puree. Cook everything in the oven for 20 minutes, until the puree is crispy.

PANCAKES WITH BERRIES & WHIPPED CREAM

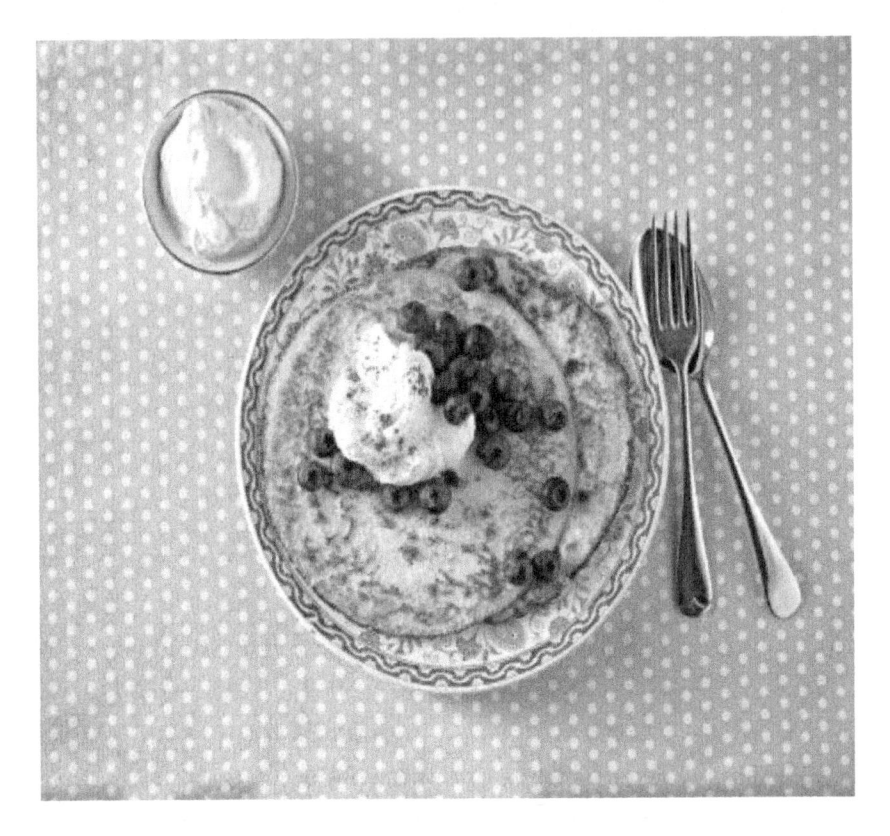

Pancakes always go! How about a low carbohydrate version with berries and whipped cream? You should try this!

Servings: 1

Preparation time: 5 minutes

Cooking time: 10 mins

Nutritional Fact: Carbohydrates: 3g

INGREDIENTS

- 2 eggs
- 2 tablespoons cream cheese
- ¼ teaspoon sweetener
- 1 pinch of cinnamon
- 40 g blueberries
- 20 ml of cream double

PREPARATION

1. Mix the eggs, cream cheese, sweetener and cinnamon to the dough. Stir the ingredients till you have a smooth dough. Let the mass rest for 2 minutes to allow the bubbles to settle.
2. Put half of the dough in a hot non-stick skillet that has been greased with butter. Fry the dough for 3 - 4 minutes over medium heat until it is golden brown, then turn over and fry for 3 minutes on the other side. Repeat this with the remaining dough. Beat the creme double until it is firm and serve the pancakes with the crème and blueberries.

SAUSAGES STUFFED MUSHROOMS

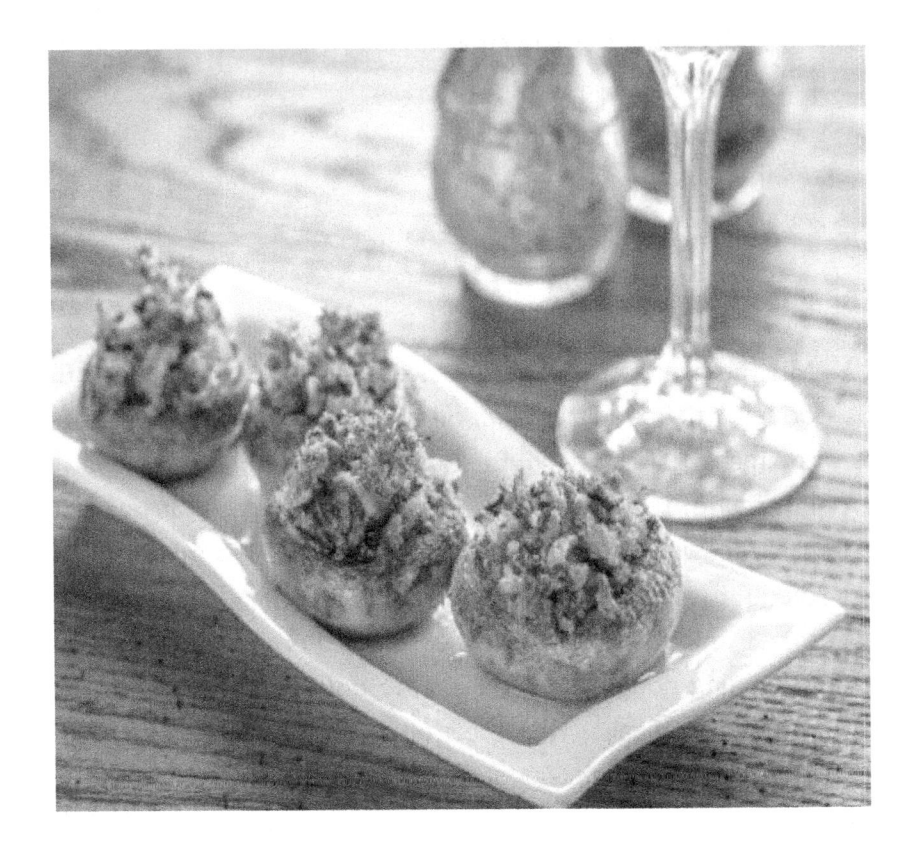

Servings: 1

Preparation time: 10 mins

Cooking time: 25 minutes

Nutritional Fact: Carbohydrates:6g

INGREDIENTS

- 2 sausages

- 1 clove of garlic
- 2 tablespoons cream cheese
- 1 tablespoon of ground flaxseed
- 1/2 onion
- Share page

PREPARATION

1. Remove the intestines and fry the sausage with the pressed garlic. Then place it on the page for later. Then remove the stems of mushrooms and chop them small. Mix the finely chopped champignon stems with the cream cheese and then add the cooled sausage meat. Finally, add the ground flax seeds and fill the mushrooms with the mixture. Place the mushrooms in a large casserole dish and bake at 160 ° C for 25 minutes.

SALMON WITH AVOCADO SALSA

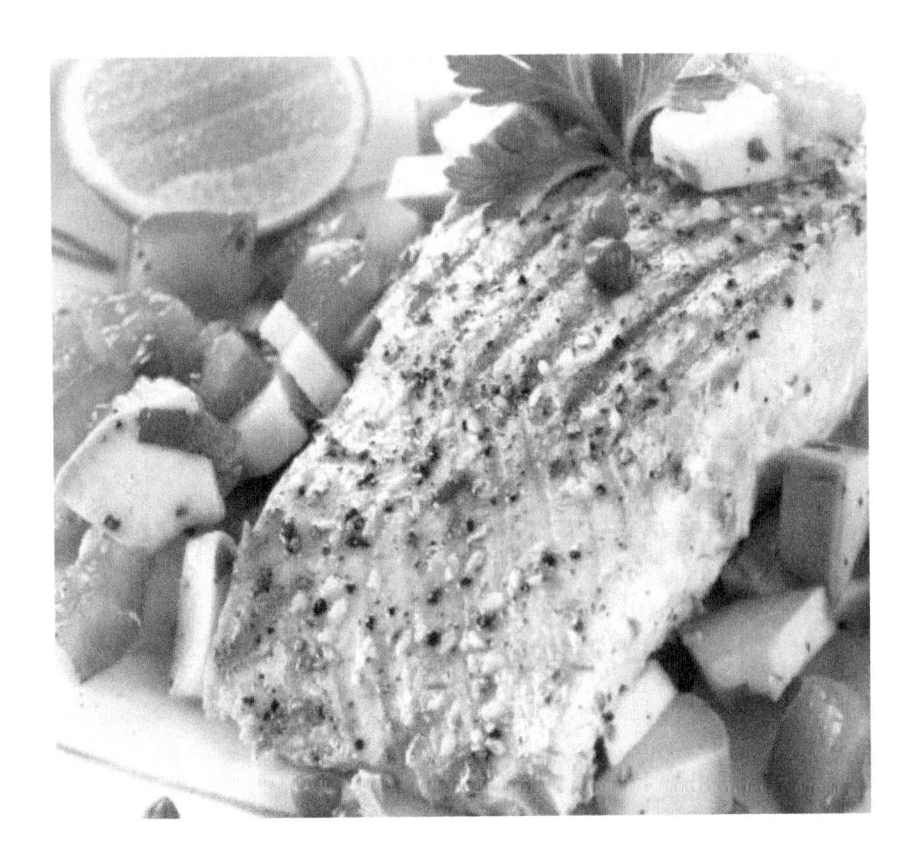

Servings: 1

Preparation time: 10 mins

Cooking time: 15 minutes

Nutritional Fact: Carbohydrates: 5g

INGREDIENTS

- 0.5 tablespoon olive oil

- 0.25 teaspoon salt
- 0.5 teaspoon black pepper
- 0.5 teaspoon paprika powder
- 115 grams of salmon fillet
- 0.5 Avocado
- 0.25 red onions
- 1 tablespoon of fresh lime juice
- 1 tablespoon of fresh coriander
- 3 cherry tomatoes

PREPARATION

2. Mix the oil, salt, pepper including paprika into a bowl. Coat the salmon fillet including the marinade and put it in the fridge for 30 minutes. Grate the salmon on both sides for two minutes over high heat.
3. Mix the avocado, chopped tomatoes, 1/4 red onion, the juice of a lime, 1 tablespoon of olive oil and salt to taste in a separate bowl. Serve the salmon on the avocado salsa and garnish with chopped cilantro. Serve with a mixed green salad.

BRIE & CARAMELIZED ONION BURGER

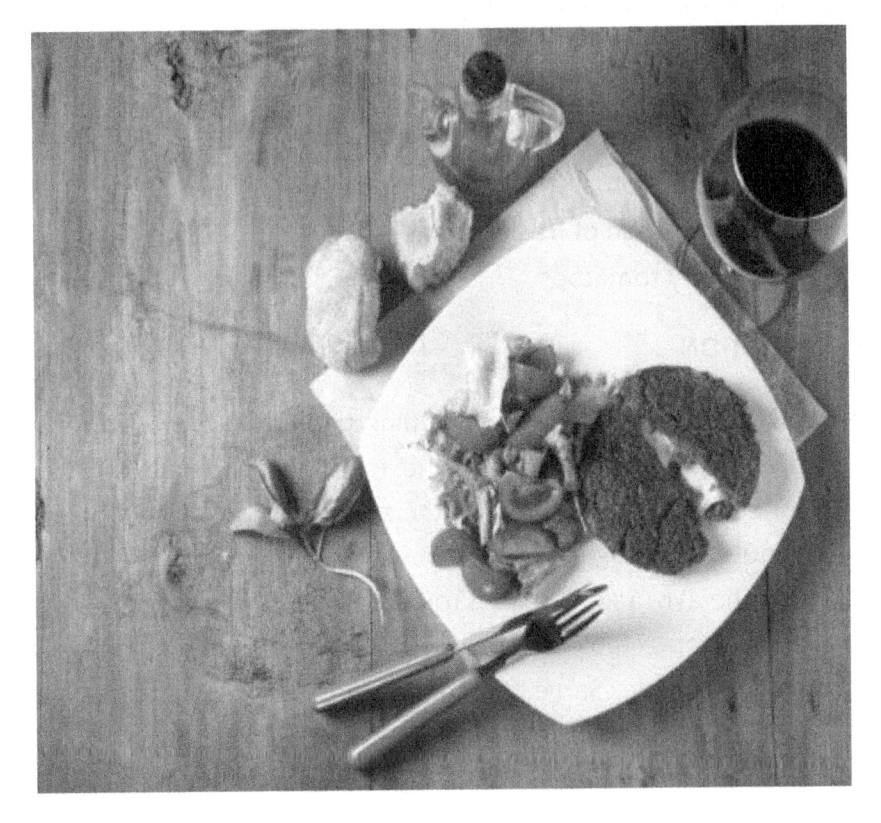

Have a low carb burger including brie and caramelized onion. A low carbohydrate burger does not have the carbohydrates (bread), but even you can enjoy the delicious taste even more!

Servings: 1

Preparation time: 10 mins

Cooking time: 20 minutes

Nutritional Fact: Carbohydrates: 5g

INGREDIENTS

- 1 tablespoon of olive oil
- 50 grams of white onion
- 1 teaspoon salt
- 1 tablespoon butter
- 3 mushrooms
- 120 grams of ground beef
- 1 teaspoon of black pepper
- 30 grams of Brie

PREPARATION

1. Preheat the grill for medium oven heat. Heat the olive oil on a large pan and fry the onions with a pinch of salt for 5 minutes until they are soft and golden brown. Do not let them get too crispy! Put the onions upon a plate for later and keep the pan handy to fry the mushrooms. Put the ground beef, salt, and pepper for the burgers in a large bowl. Knead the mass well by hand and form 2 patties. Cover one half with a bit of brie and onions, then put the second half on top of the cheese plus onions to form the burger! Put the burgers under a preheated grill and grill each side for 4-5 minutes. While the burgers are grilling, fry the mushrooms in a little butter for 2 - 3 minutes. Once the burgers are cooked, take them off the grill.

BEEF AND BROCCOLI PAN

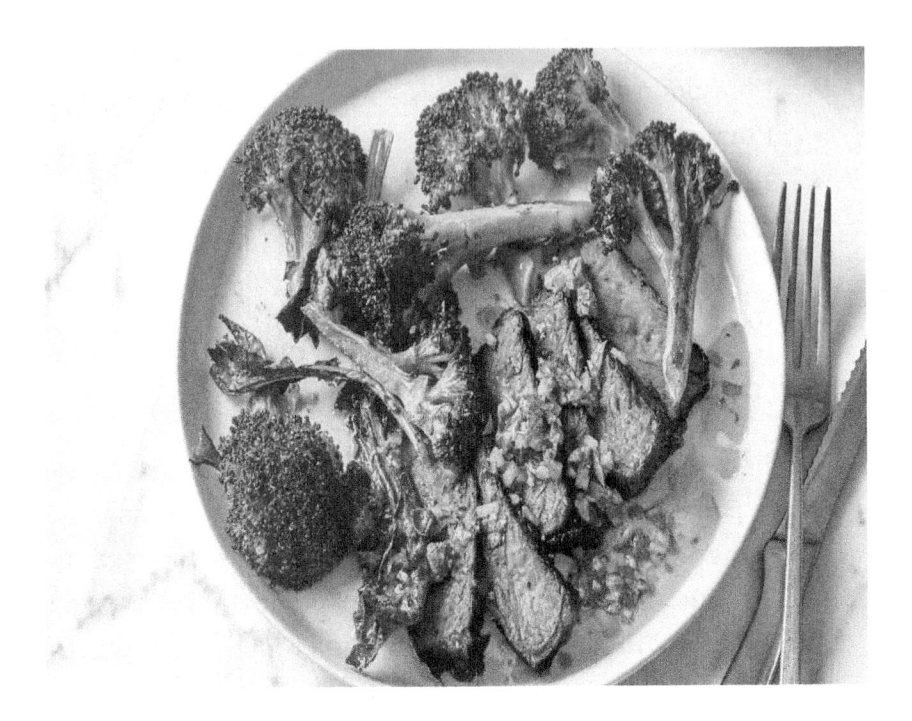

The mixture of beef and broccoli is not simply healthy but also a great choice when it comes to carbohydrates. This dish has only 6 grams of carbohydrates and tons of protein and vitamins!

Servings: 2

Preparation time: 15 minutes

Cooking time: 30 minutes

Carbohydrates: 6g

INGREDIENTS

- 100 grams of broccoli
- 150 grams of beef, high-quality steak
- 1 tablespoon soy sauce
- 1 clove of garlic
- 1 tablespoon of oil
- 30 ml of water
- ½ tablespoon of fresh ginger
- ½ teaspoon of red pepper flakes
- 1 tablespoon of apple cider vinegar
- 100 ml beef broth
- 1/2 red chili pepper
- 1/2 tablespoon sesame seeds

PREPARATION

1. Cut the washed broccoli into small florets and the stems into long strips. Put the chopped broccoli aside.
2. Cut the beef into strips about 0.5 cm thick. In a bowl, mix the beef with the soy sauce and garlic and let it simmer for 15 minutes in the marinade. Prepare the sauce by mixing the broth, apple cider vinegar, red pepper flakes, and ginger.
3. Place the pan on the stove with a tablespoon of oil over medium heat. If the oil is hot, add half of the meat mixture and fry for about 2 minutes until the meat is through. Bring it out of the pan and set it aside. Add another tbsp of oil and fry the remaining meat.
4. Pour the remaining oil into the pan. Once the oil is hot, add the broccoli and chili and cook for about 1 minute. Add water, cover the pan and stir until the broccoli is cooked

about 3 minutes. Add the sauce and meat. Cook until the sauce boils and reduces. Put the pan on a plate and garnish with sesame seeds.

POTATO AND PUMPKIN SALAD

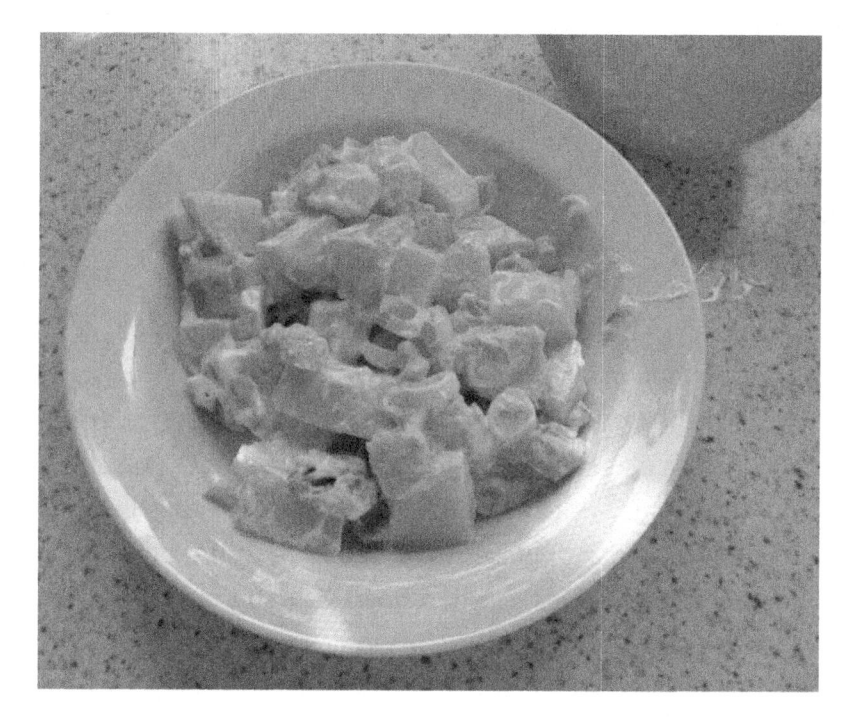

Potatoes, pumpkin, and pecans make this recipe for a potato pumpkin salad a special taste experience.

25 min. Total time

25 min. preparation time

INGREDIENTS for 6 servings

- 500G   pumpkin
- 560G   potatoes
- 6 stk   spring onions
- 40G   pecans

- 3 stg   celery
- 12:25   cup   parsley
- 0.5 cup   mayonnaise
- 75 G   sour cream
- 1 TL   Dijon mustard
- 1 prize   Pepper, freshly ground

PREPARATION

1. Peel the pumpkin, take out the seeds, then chop into small pieces with the peeled potatoes and then cook gently. Strain and allow cooling.
2. Slice the spring onions into thin rings, cut the celery into small cubes and finely chop the parsley. Put all the ingredients with the pumpkin and the potatoes in a salad bowl. Mix mayonnaise, sour cream, mustard including and the pepper inside a small bowl. Stir the marinade under the salad.

VEGETABLE RAGOUT

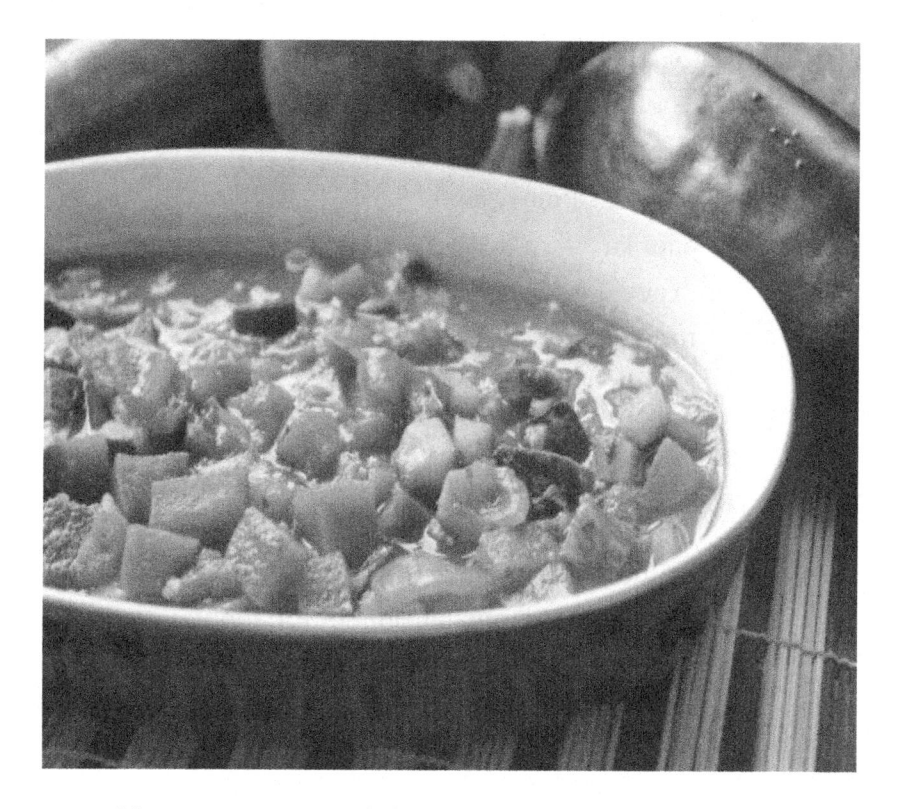

Vegetable ragout tastes delicious and is healthy. This recipe is served cold.

90 min. Total time

40 min. Preparation time

50 min. cooking time

INGREDIENTS for 8 servings

- 500 G eggplant

- 1 prize salt
- 2 stk red peppers
- 500 G zucchini
- 2 stk big onions
- 4 stk Garlic cloves
- 100 ml olive oil
- 2 TL ground cumin
- 1 TL paprika
- 1msp cayenne pepper
- 4stk tomatoes
- 1stk Lemon, juice
- 4 EL chopped coriander

PREPARATION

2. Wash the aubergines, remove the stalks, dice them, place in a sieve, sprinkle with salt and let simmer for about 30 minutes.
3. Wash the peppers, halve, core and cut into small cubes. Wash the zucchini; remove from the stalks, and dice small. Peel the onions and finely chop. Peel the garlic and then squeeze it through a garlic press.
4. Preheat oven to 200 ° C - 170 ° C, preheat gas to stage 3. Dab the eggplant cubes dry. Put the prepared vegetables with garlic, olive oil, and the spices into a casserole and mix well. Cook the whole on the middle rack in the oven for about 30 minutes.
5. Wash the tomatoes, cut in half, remove from the stalk, remove seeds and dice. Add the tomato cubes to the cooked vegetable mixture after 30 minutes. Cook for another 20 minutes in the oven.
6. Add the lemon juice and cilantro to the vegetables. Mix everything and let it cool.

CANNELLONI WITH RICOTTA, SPINACH, AND ZUCCHINI

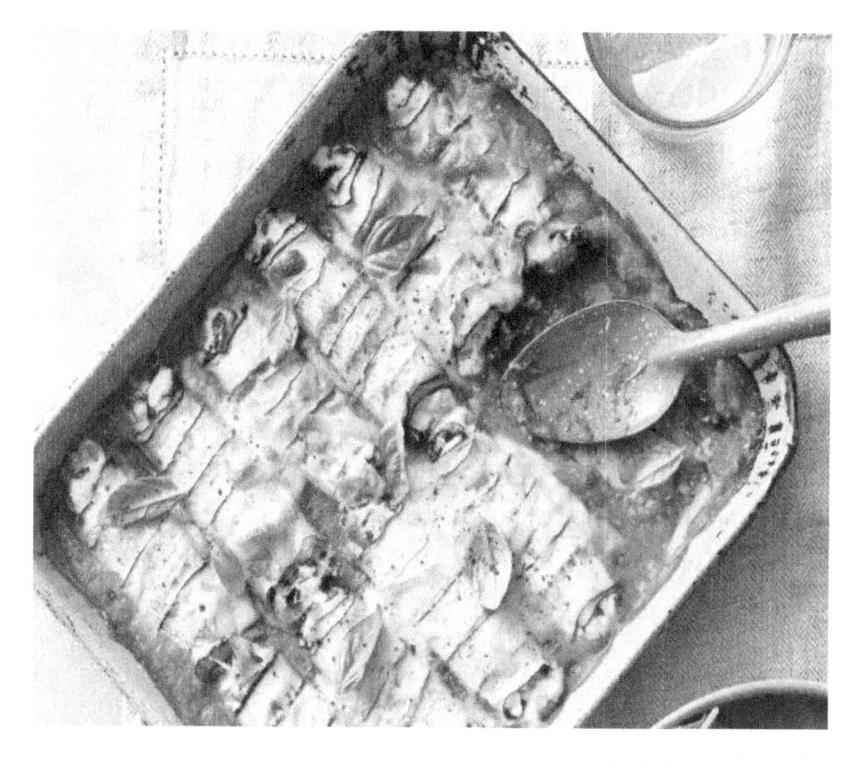

Low-carbohydrate zucchini instead of "real" cannelloni ensure that even low carb fans will be happy with this delicious casserole. Tomato puree provides us with lycopene, an antioxidant that protects our cells from damage. Ricotta and mozzarella not only increase the protein content of the delicious dish, but also provide plenty of bone-strengthening calcium.

Preparation: 25 min

Calories: 591 kcal

INGREDIENTS

- 4 Big zucchini (1.2 kg)
- 100 g Spinach
- 100 g Chard
- Salt
- 1 Clove of garlic
- ½ bunches
- Basil (10 g)
- 450 g Ricotta (45% fat)
- 1 Egg yolk
- ½ Organic lemons (shell)
- Pepper
- 2 tsps. Olive oil
- 500 g Tomato purees (glass)
- 1 Tsp. Dried Italian herbs
- Two balls Mozzarella (250 g)
- One piece Parmesan (40 g, 30% fat)

PREPARATION

1. Clean the zucchini wash and cut into thin slices. Clean spinach and chard, wash, remove from coarse stems and cook in boiling salted water for about 2 minutes. Then drain, chill off cold, express well and chop roughly. Peel garlic and chop finely. Wash the basil, shake dry, peel off the leaves, put aside some for the garnish, finely chop the rest.
2. Put the ricotta inside a bowl and mix with garlic, egg yolk, lemon peel, chopped basil, spinach and chard, season with salt and pepper.
3. Brush an ovenproof dish with one teaspoon of olive oil. Season the tomato puree with salt, pepper, and Italian herbs and place half in the mold. Layout 3-4 zucchini slices

overlapping each other on a work surface, add 2 tbsps. of ricotta and vegetable stuffing and roll up. Place the zucchini cannelloni with the seam down on the sauce in the mold. Spread the remaining tomato puree all around and spread over it.

4. Chop the mozzarella, grate the parmesan. Sprinkle the cannelloni and tomato puree with the cheese, drizzle with remaining oil and bake in a pre-heated oven or deep fryer at 200 ° C (180 ° C convection, gas: level 3) for about 30-35 minutes until the cheese is melted and slightly browned. Remove and spread the remaining basil leaves over the cannelloni.

CHICKEN MELON SALAD

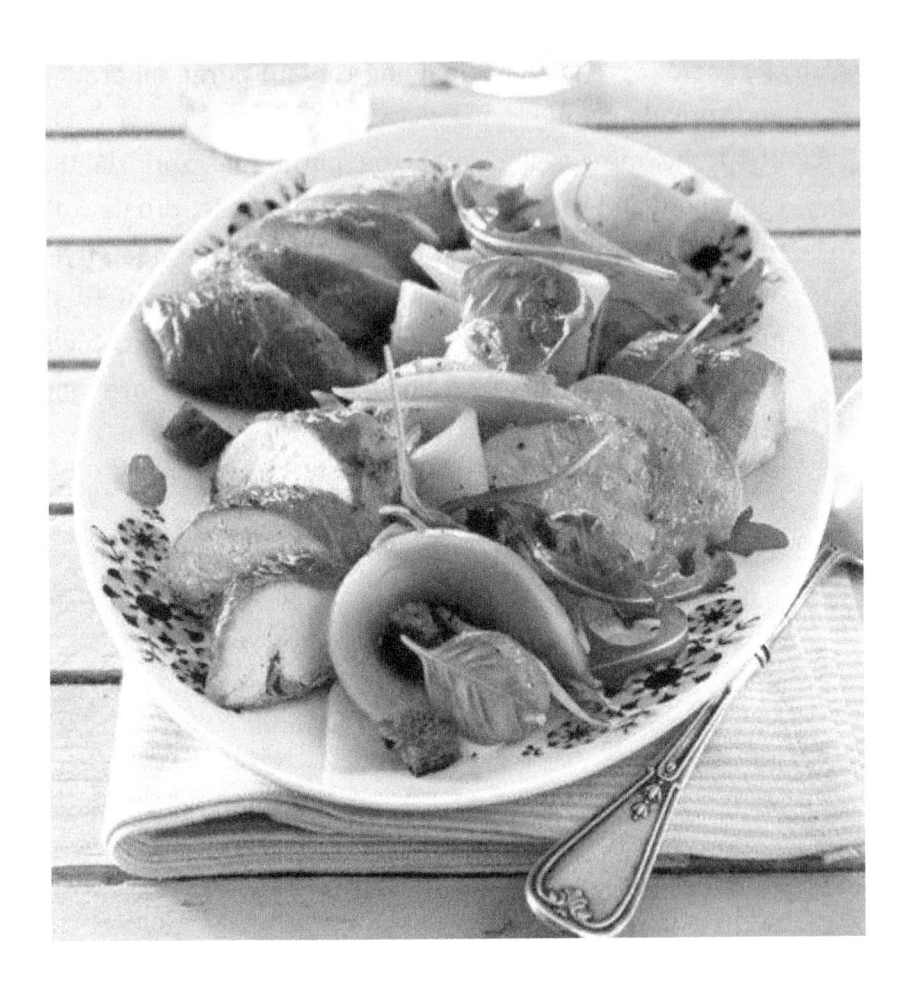

INGREDIENTS for four servings

- Two slices of mixed rye bread
- Four tablespoons olive oil
- Four chicken fillets (approx. 150 g each)
- Salt
- Pepper

- Eight slices of Parma ham (approx. 15 g each)
- ½ cantaloupe melon
- Three tablespoons light balsamic vinegar
- 1 - 2 tablespoons of liquid honey
- One bunch of rocket
- Five stems of basil

PREPARATION

1. Dice the bread, fry in 1 tablespoon of oil until crispy. Drain on kitchen paper.
2. Salt meat and pepper, wrap with two slices of ham. Heat 1 tablespoon of oil in an oven-proof pan. Sauté the chicken briefly, cook in the hot oven (cooker: 200 C / circulating air 175 ° C) for about 8 minutes.
3. Meanwhile, cut the melon into thin slices. Season 2 tablespoons of oil with vinegar and honey, season. Mix dressing with rocket, melon, croutons, and basil.

Per serving about 450 kcal

ZUCCHINI WITH YOGURT DIP

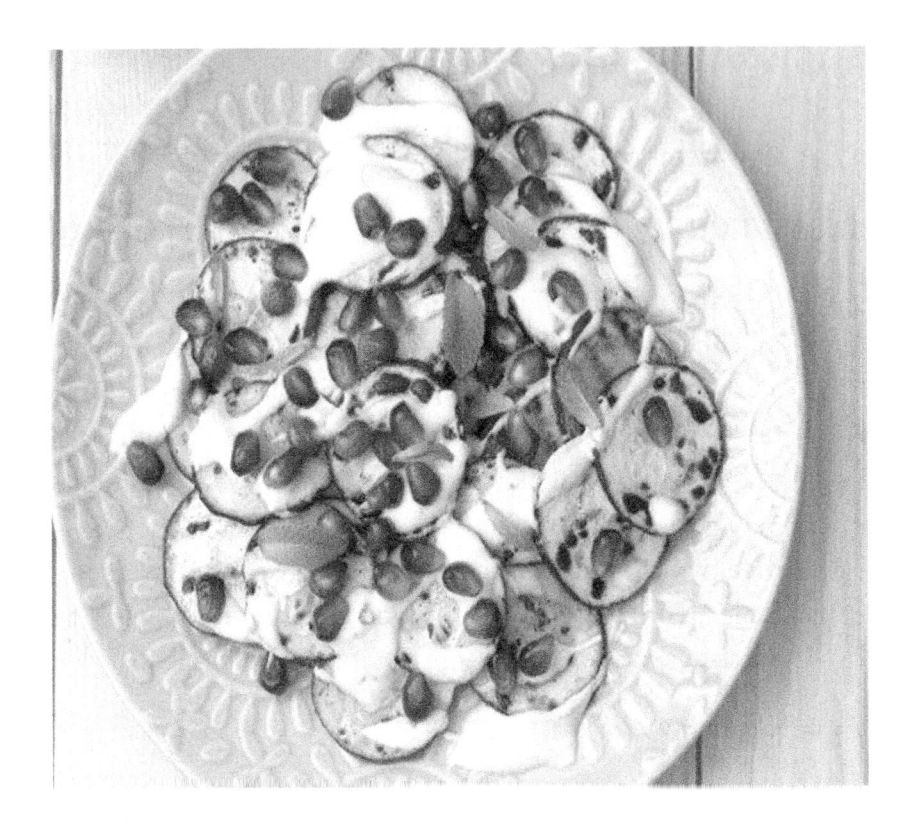

Preparation: 25 min

Calories: 193 kcal

Zucchini contains around 90% water as well as hematopoietic iron and nerve-strengthening magnesium. Yogurt, with its lactic acid bacteria, soothes the intestines and promotes digestion.

INGREDIENTS

- For four portions

- Three zucchini (700 g)
- 2 tbsps. olive oil
- ½ lemons (juice)
- Salt
- Pepper
- One handful mint (5 g)
- 1 tsp. sambal oelek
- 500 g yogurt (1.5% fat)
- One pomegranate (250 g)

PREPARATION

1. Clean, wash and slice the zucchini. Mix the zucchini slices with oil and lemon juice and season with salt and pepper.
2. Heat a grill pan. Fry the zucchini in slices on both sides for 2-3 minutes over medium heat.
3. Wash mint, shake dry, peel off leaves, put aside some for garnish. Chop the rest for the dip and stir in the yogurt with Sambal oelek, then season with one pinch of salt and pepper.
4. Halve the pomegranate and then remove the seeds from the fruit. Arrange the zucchini slices on plates and drizzle with the yogurt dip. Spread the pomegranate seeds over them and garnish with mint leaves.

ROMAINE LETTUCE WITH RADISHES AND AVOCADO YOGURT SAUCE

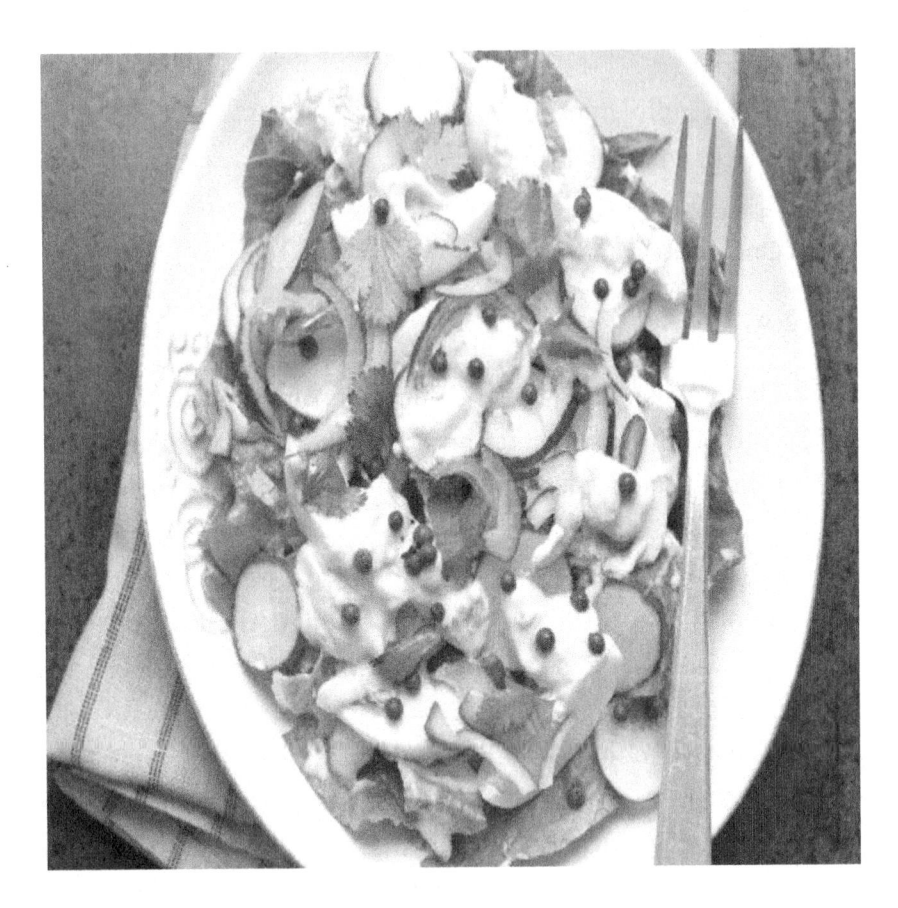

Preparation: 35 min

Calories: 177 kcal

Due to its lactic acid bacteria, yogurt has a beneficial effect on the intestine and promotes digestion. Also, the dairy product is rich in calcium and a good source of protein. With the high-fat avocado, good fats, lots of potassium and vitamin E are in the salad.

INGREDIENTS

- For four portions
- Two green peppers
- 1 tbsp. white wine vinegar
- 1 tbsp. olive oil
- Four eggs
- ½ clove of garlic
- One lime
- ¼ ripe avocados (50 g)
- 200 g yogurt (0.3% fat)
- Some splash of Worcester sauce
- Salt
- Pepper
- One head romaine lettuce (300 g)
- One red onion
- One bunch radish
- ½ bunch coriander (10 g)
- 2 tsp. Pickled green pepper (or glass, 10 g)

PREPARATION

1. Cut the peppers into half, corer them, wash it and grill with the skin side up in the preheated oven with the grill function until the paprika skin is black. Then allow cooling slightly. Peel off the skin, finely chop the pepper and marinate with vinegar and olive oil for about 15 minutes.
2. Meanwhile, boil eggs in 8-10 minutes. Then put off, peel and cut into slices.
3. In the meantime peel garlic for the sauce and finely chop. Halve the lime and squeeze juice. Remove the core of the avocado and lift the flesh out of the shell. Puree garlic, lime

juice, avocado, yogurt and Worcester sauce with a hand blender. Season the sauce with salt and pepper.
4. Clean the lettuce, wash, cut into small pieces and spin dry. Peel the onion, halve and cut into strips. Clean radishes, wash and slice them. Wash cilantro, shake dry and peel off leaves.
5. Mix salad with diced peppers and serve on plates. Spread onions, eggs and radishes on top. Drizzle with the sauce spread the green pepper and garnish with coriander leaves.

MONKFISH AND SPINACH PARCELS

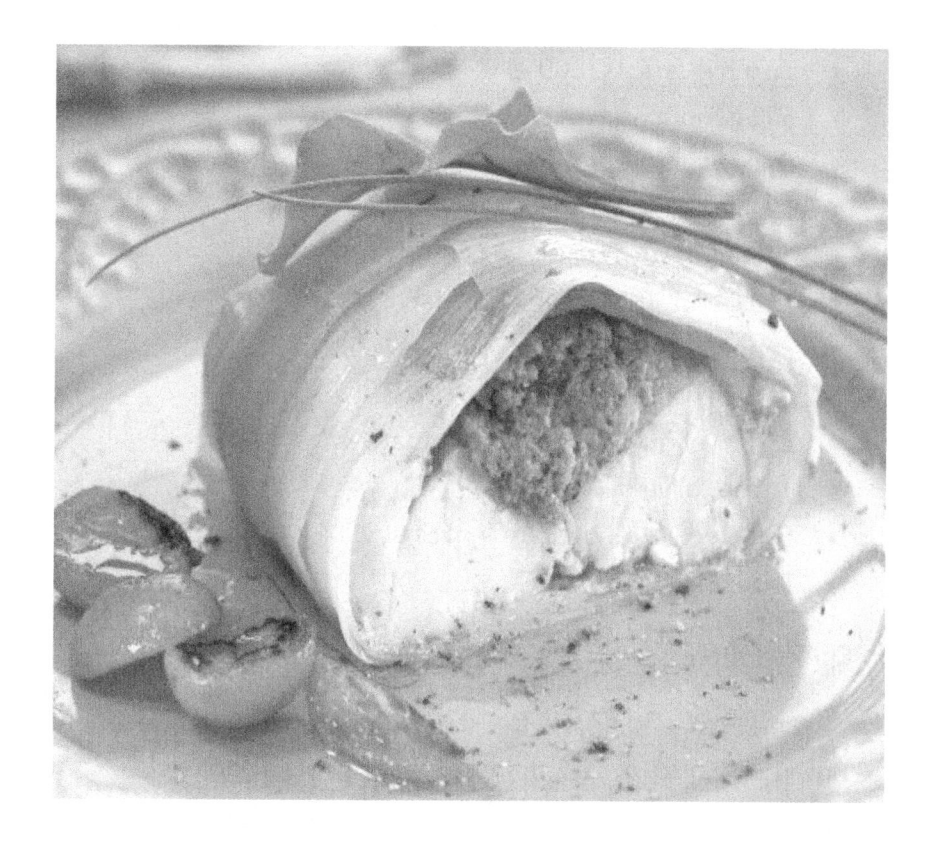

Preparation: 45 min

Calories: 351 kcal

The sea fish provides plenty of iodine and protein. Both ensure a smooth flow of metabolism. The spicy-tasting leek is very rich in zinc and thus has a wound-healing an immune-boosting effect.

Ingredients

- For four portions

- 50 g spinach
- Salt
- 2 bars leek
- Two big carrots (300 g)
- 600 g monkfish
- One organic lemon
- 300 g seelachsfilet
- 100 ml of soy cream
- 150 g cottage cheese (0.3% fat)
- Pepper
- 100 ml fish stock (glass)
- 250 g yellow or red cherry tomatoes
- 1 tbsp. olive oil
- Four red sorrel orchard leaves at will
- ¼ bunch chives (5 g)

PREPARATION

1. Clean, wash, and drizzle the spinach in boiling salted water and let it collapse in 1-2 minutes. Remove spinach, chill cold, squeeze well, chop and chill.
2. Clean the leeks cut in length and wash. Separate the leaves from each other and add to the boiling salted water for 2 minutes. Then remove cold quench and dab dry.
3. Clean and peel the carrots, cut lengthways into thin strips, and add to the boiling salted water for 3 minutes until soft. Remove, chill off cold and dab carrot strips dry.
4. Wash monkfish fillet and pat dry. Lay the bottom of an ovenproof mold slightly overlapping with the leek and carrot strips. Place the monkfish filet in the middle of it.
5. Rinse the lemon hot, rub dry, rub the skin, and squeeze the juice. Cut the salmon filet into small pieces and puree with soy

cream, cottage cheese and spinach to a fine mass. Season the mixture with salt, pepper, lemon peel, and the juice, spread on the fillet and beat the vegetable strips over the fish from both sides.
6. Add fish stock and cook the monkfish fillet in a preheated oven at 180 ° C (160 ° C convection, gas: stage 2-3) for about 30 minutes.
7. In the meantime wash and halve cherry tomatoes. In a frying pan, fry the tomatoes in it for about 5 minutes over medium heat.
8. Wash lettuce leaves and chives and shake dry. Cut monkfish fillet in leek and carrot clove into four pieces and arrange with tomatoes, lettuce leaves, and chives.

CHICKEN BREAST WITH AVOCADO AND CAULIFLOWER MASH

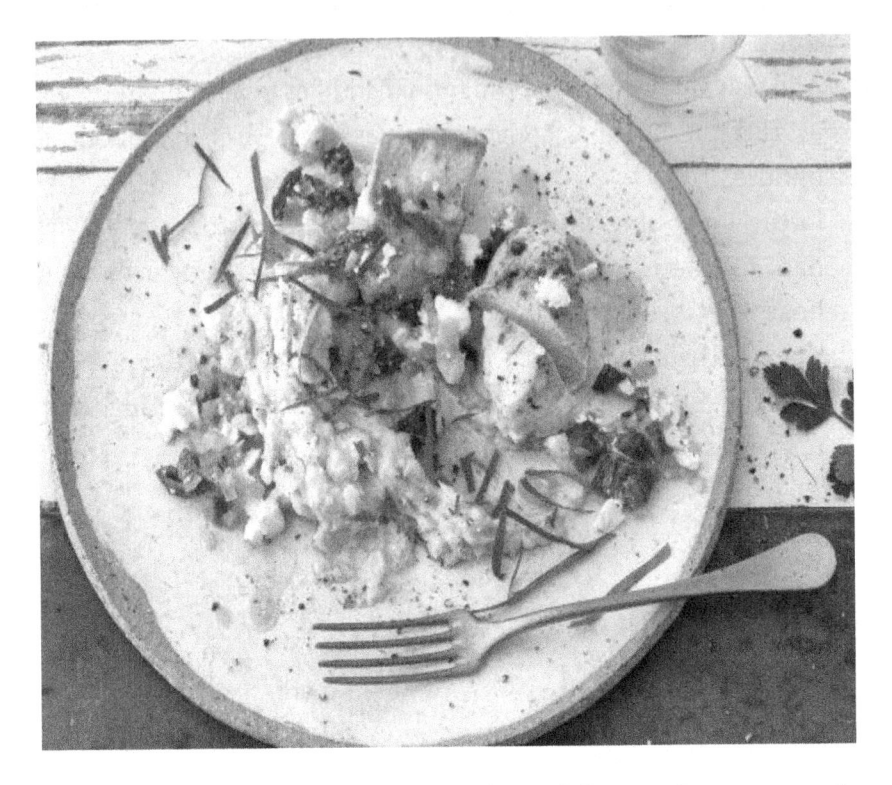

Chicken Breast with Avocado and Cauliflower Stomp, tender poultry with an aromatic side dish just delicious and made fast!

Preparation: 25 min

Calories: 294 kcal

Although the avocado is high in calories and high in fat, it is excellent for fasting because it has plenty of vitamin E, potassium and good fats. The tender chicken provides plenty of protein; the cheese contains a lot of bone-strengthening calcium.

INGREDIENTS

- For four portions
- ½ cauliflowers (600 g)
- Salt
- One onion
- 50 g sun-dried tomatoes
- 2 tbsps. rapeseed oil
- Pepper
- Four chicken breast fillets (à 125 g)
- Three tbsps. lemon juice
- 80 ml milk (3.5% fat)
- 80 ml of vegetable stock
- ½ ripe avocado
- 80 g feta (9% fat)
- Chives tip

PREPARATION

1. Clean and wash the cauliflower, divide into florets and cook gently in a little salted water over medium heat for 8-10 minutes. Then drain.
2. Meanwhile, peel and dice the onion. Cut tomatoes in small pieces, little heat oil in a pan, sauté onions and tomatoes for 2 minutes over medium heat. Salt, pepper, and remove from the pan.
3. Rinse chicken breast fillets, pat dry, salt and pepper, heat remaining oil in the pan. Fry the meat on both sides for 5-8 minutes over medium heat. Sprinkle with lemon juice and remove the pan from the heat; Cover the meat and let it spread.

4. Warm milk with broth, remove the core from the avocado and lift the pulp out of the shell. Cauliflower and avocado meat in a bowl, mash with a fork, mix in the warm milk stock and season with salt and pepper.
5. Spread the stomping on plates for serving and put the chicken breast on top. Sprinkle onion-tomato mixture, crumble feta and spread over it. Garnish with chives and sprinkle with pepper as you like.

CHILI BEEF PAN

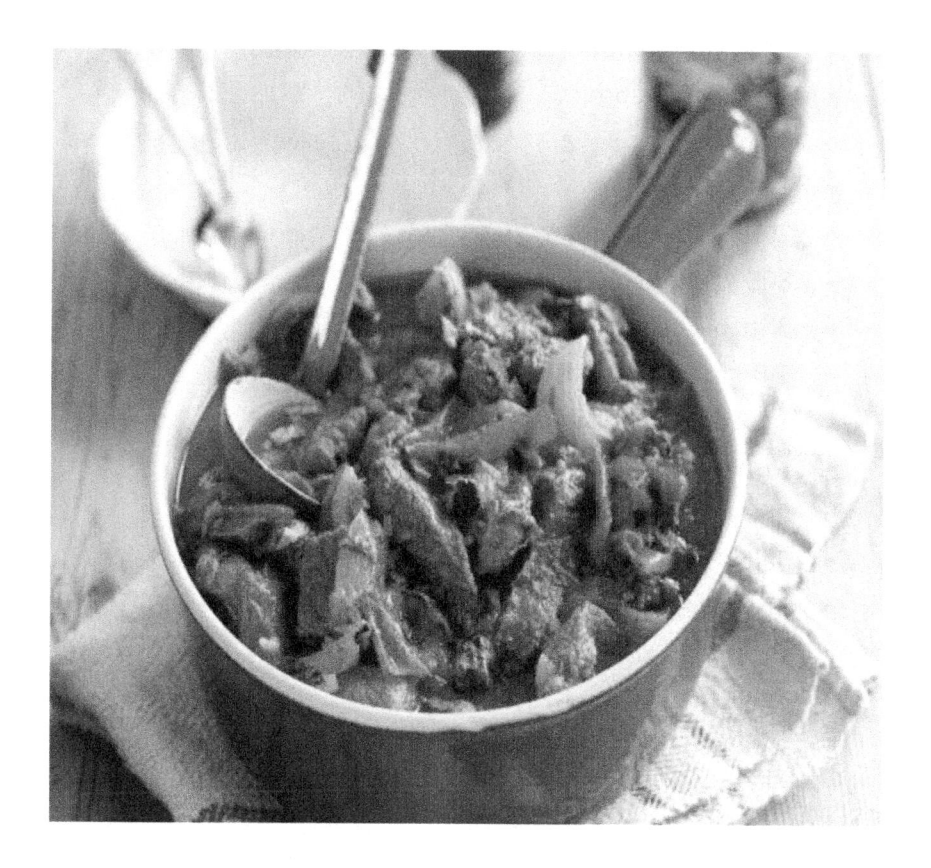

Preparation: 15 minutes

Finished in 55 min

Calories: 450 kcal

Beef contains a lot of protein as well as large amounts of iron. The trace element it needs among other things for blood formation. Peppers score with immune-boosting vitamin C; the tomatoes deliver cell-protecting lycopene.

INGREDIENTS

- For 4 portions
- 6 pointed pepper (yellow and red)
- 1 red chili pepper
- 1 onion
- 1 clove of garlic
- 200 g cherry tomatoes
- 800 g lean beef (e.g. rump steak)
- 3 tbsps. olive oil
- 1 tbsp. tomato paste (20 g)
- 2 tbsps.
- Noble sweet paprika powder
- 750 ml of meat soup
- Salt
- Pepper
- Ground Coriander
- Ground caraway
- ½ bunch parsley (10 g)

PREPARATION

1. Wash peppers, clean and cut into strips. Wash, clean and finely chop the chili pepper. Peel onion and garlic. Finely chop the onion and finely chop garlic. Wash, clean and halve tomatoes.
2. Dab meat dries with kitchen paper and cuts into bite-sized strips. Then heat a little oil in a pan and sauté the meat in portions over high heat for 2-3 minutes. Take it out of the pan.
3. Pure one tbsp. of oil into the pan, and then sauté the chili, onion, and then add garlic over medium heat. Add the

tomato puree and paprika powder and sauté for 1 minute. Pour broth, add meat, paprika and tomatoes and season with salt, pepper, coriander, and cumin. Simmer over minimum heat for about 35 minutes. Stir in between and add some broth if necessary.
4. Meanwhile, wash parsley, shake dry and chop. Season the pepper-beef pan with salt and pepper, sprinkle with parsley and serve immediately.

STEAMED COD

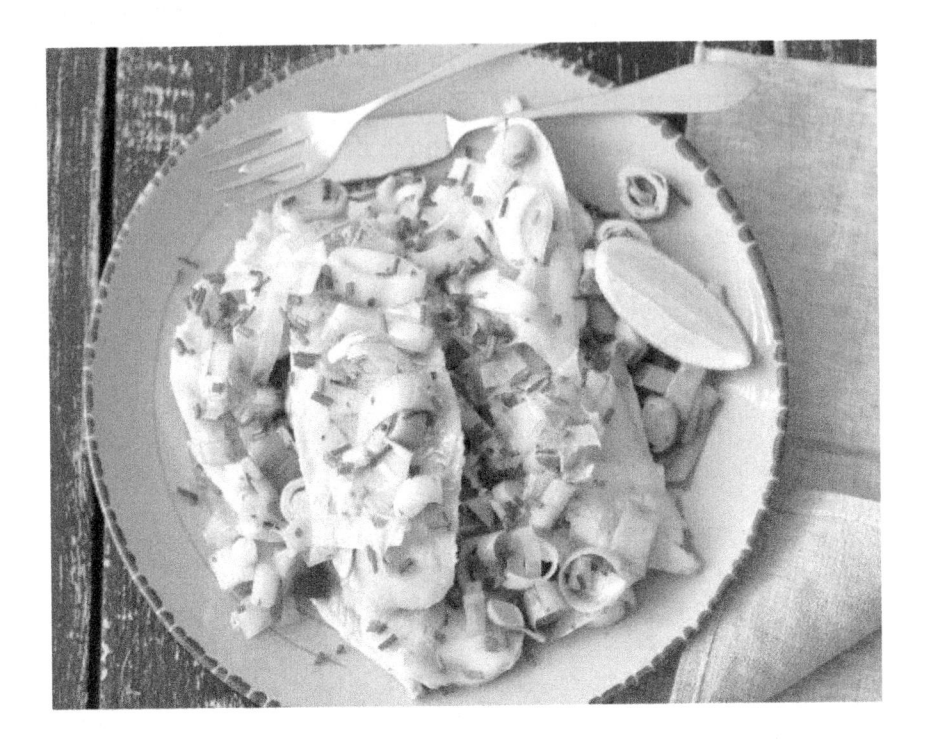

Preparation: 30 min

Calories: 226 kcal

The high-quality protein in the cod stimulates the metabolism and serves as a building material for cells, muscles, enzymes, and hormones. Valuable proteins also prevent cravings and muscle breakdown.

INGREDIENTS

- For four portions
- Four cod fillets (à 150 g)

- 4 tbsps. lemon juice
- 2 bars leek
- 3 tbsps. rapeseed oil
- 100 ml of vegetable stock
- salt
- pepper
- ½ dried thyme
- ½ bunch chives (10 g)
- One organic lemon

PREPARATION

1. Rinse the fish fillets, pat dry and drizzle with 2 tbsps. lemon juice. Clean leeks, wash and cut into rings.
2. Heat 1 tbsps. Oil in a pan, dab fish dry, sauté for 2 minutes at medium heat. Then turn over, add the remaining lemon juice and 50 ml of vegetable stock and cover, cook for 5-7 minutes on low heat.
3. Meanwhile, heat remaining oil in a saucepan, sauté the leek rings in medium heat for 2 minutes, season with salt, pepper, and thyme. Add remaining vegetable stock and cook the leek for 5 minutes over low heat.
4. Meanwhile, wash chives, shake dry and cut into small rolls. Rinse lemon hot and cut into quarters.
5. Season fish fillets and leeks with salt and pepper, arrange on plates and garnish with chives and lemon quarters.

FOR WHOM IS THE ATKINS DIET SUITABLE?

- For healthy, adult people, this diet is suitable.
- If you suffer from kidney or liver damage, you should rather do without such a protein diet.
- Even children or young people who are still growing, the diet is not recommended because many nutrients are important, which are important for development.
- For diabetics, however, it is a good alternative, since, in the diet, very little insulin is released.
- Very seriously overweight people should consult a doctor beforehand and have their blood values checked so that a health risk can be ruled out.
- Also, the Atkins diet is not for vegans or vegetarians, as the main ingredient of the diet are meat and animal products.

HOW INDIVIDUAL IS THE ATKINS DIET?

- For all dieters, the same rules and quantities apply. So you are not individually tailored to the individual.
- Due to the high protein content of animal products, this form of diet is not adaptable to special eating habits such as vegetarianism or veganism.

How flexible is the Atkins diet?

- There is no annoying calorie counting needed, and it must be dispensed quasi only on carbohydrates. Thus, this diet is also feasible for, eg, working people.
- No special food is needed, and a restaurant visit is no obstacle. One should do without carbohydrate-rich side dishes.

How suitable is the Atkins diet for everyday use?

- The complete abandonment of carbohydrates makes the diet quite one-sided
- Even eating out can be a problem from time to time. On the other hand, one has free choice among the allowed recipes and is not limited in the amount

How scientific is the Atkins diet?

- The success of the Atkins diet is detectable, but this is mainly due to the calorie reduction itself and not to the renunciation of carbohydrates.
- The drastic renouncement of carbohydrates is to be regarded critically since carbohydrates are the number one energy supplier for the body. So when you completely erase them from the diet, the body is forced to draw energy from muscle mass and fat. This also suffers the muscles underneath, and it can lead to muscle cramps.
- The high protein content in the diet is bad for the body in the long term. Not only does the insulin level increase, but a portion of uric acid accumulates during the division and digestion of proteins. If the protein intake is too high, the toxic substance can be deposited in the kidney and cause lasting damage. A long-term consequence can even be cardiovascular disease.

How Sustainable Is The Atkins Diet, And What Are Its Risks?

- Keeping strictly to the rules and rules of the diet, you can achieve quick results, especially in the early stages. The later stages then serve to acclimatize and adapt, so that the weight can be kept.
- However, this type of diet can / should not be maintained permanently because, due to the high proportion of animal fats, health risks are not ruled out and fatigue and impairment of the immune system can occur in the long term due to the high carbohydrate deficiency.

- The weight reduction happens very fast and not necessarily sustainable, which is why the risk of succumbing to the yo-yo effect after ending the diet is quite high.
- The principle of the Atkins diet relies on ketosis: In the absence of carbohydrates for energy metabolism, fatty acids in the liver are converted into ketone bodies to ensure energy readiness.
- However, this also carries the risk of increased triglyceride levels. Highly obese people, as well as diabetics or people who suffer from a lipid metabolism disease, usually already suffer from an increased triglyceride value anyway. The consequence of this is an increased risk of thrombosis.
- Also, the often mentioned extreme carbohydrate deficiency could lead to any amount of deficiency symptoms. Symptoms of this include fatigue, muscle cramps, high cholesterol, and lipid levels, kidney and liver damage, or even high blood pressure.

Method

To achieve effective customer success with the Atkins diet, the diet seeker should follow the four-step model: At the beginning of the phases, the goal is to limit the consumption of carbohydrates. During the subsequent phases, the declining person is slowly brought back to the consumption of carbohydrates. In the first phase of the Atkins diet, also known as the "induction phase," no more than 20 grams of carbohydrates should be ingested daily for two weeks. To calculate the exact amount of carbohydrates, calculators, and scales can be used.

Furthermore, there are numerous carbohydrate tables, from which the values can be easily read. All other foods, however, are allowed without limitation. The subsequent reduction phase already allows more carbohydrates. In the beginning week of the second phase, the carbohydrate amount is increased by five grams. This will be continued week after week until further weight reduction takes place. During this phase, the critical amount of carbohydrate is approached. The critical amount of carbohydrates is the number of carbohydrates that you continue to lose weight with. If one realizes that no weight reduction takes place, the daily amount of carbohydrates should be screwed down again. Since the Atkins diet does not include a balanced diet, dietary supplements should be used during the second phase to avoid possible deficiency symptoms.

The third phase of the diet plan should be started before reaching the target weight. It can be seen as a preparatory phase for the fourth and final phase. During this time, the daily amount of carbohydrates is increased to ten grams per week. The losers should be aware that now only a slow weight loss. If the weight reduction stops, you should go back to phase two. If the desired weight is reached, you finally reached phase four.

The fourth phase is considered to be a lifelong diet. With it, the achieved weight should be kept. It should be lived permanently according to the Atkins diet plan, which means a lot of fat and protein, little fruits and vegetables are consumed. It is important that the number of carbohydrates can always be increased until you discover more kilos on the scales again. During this time, the daily amount of carbohydrates is increased to ten grams per week. The losers should be aware that now only a slow weight loss. If the weight reduction stops, you should go back to phase two. If the desired weight is reached, you finally reached phase four.

Implementation in everyday life

The Atkins diet brings at first glance, no renunciation, only on the number of carbohydrates, should be respected. People who like to eat bread, pasta, or rice and can hardly give it up should rather choose a different diet. Even for fruit and vegetable lovers, the Atkins diet plan could be a challenge. Since no annoying calorie counting is needed, the diet can also be easily implemented for working people. However, if you plan to go on a diet with your entire family, you should choose a different diet. Especially for children who are still growing, the diet is not recommended. Because the recipes of the Atkins diet use conventional foods and do not require any extraordinary spices, can be easily bought in the familiar supermarket. Many delivery companies and restaurants are also happy to respond to the needs of their customers and leave on demand carbohydrate-side supplements easily or exchange them with others. Thus, eating out during the Atkins diet is no problem. To avoid deficiencies during diet as already mentioned dietary supplements are recommended. However, a little more money for the preparations must be included. To avoid deficiencies during diet as already mentioned dietary supplements are recommended. However, a little more money for the preparations must be included. To avoid deficiencies during diet as already mentioned dietary supplements are recommended. However, a little more money for the preparations must be included.

Scientific

Although studies prove the success of Dr. Diet's diet, Atkins, however, this is mainly due to the reduction in calorie intake. The small number of carbohydrates should be viewed critically: the brain and muscles need this nutrient. If it is supplied to the body so only slightly, it can quickly lead to unpleasant muscle spasms. The high proportion of animal fat and protein is also to be viewed critically. The cholesterol in the body can thereby be increased, which in turn can result in increased blood fat and uric acid levels. If these values are too high, the diminishing risk of developing gout or cardiovascular diseases is at risk. Atkins relies on the process of ketosis: lack of carbohydrates for energy metabolism, fatty acids in the liver are converted into ketone bodies, to ensure energy readiness. However, too much ketone formation can lead, among other things, to renal insufficiency, liver damage, constipation, hypertension, and gout, as the ketone bodies cannot be sufficiently excreted. The special diet of the Atkins diet can also increase triglyceride levels. Having too high triglyceride levels in the blood increases the risk of developing atherosclerosis and thrombosis.

In most cases, people who are overweight have diabetes or dyslipidemia already have an elevated triglyceride level anyway. Also, as the body is constantly exposed to a high intake of protein during the Atkins diet, this could put a strain on the kidneys.

Consideration of Sports

To achieve optimal weight loss, the Atkins Diet Diet Plan also includes a regular exercise program. Endurance sports such as jogging, swimming, or cycling should be run two or three times a week. Heavily overweight people should go swimming rather than jogging to protect the joints. Also, strength training is also provided. Here, too, should seriously overweight or athletic inexperienced in advance prefer to seek advice to avoid consequential damage.

Long-term effect

If you stick to the strict rules and regulations during the Atkins phases, you can expect enormous weight loss. According to the diet finder, you can already lose up to seven kilograms of weight in the first two weeks. In phase one, two and three can tumble between 0.5 to 1.5 kilograms per week. In phase four, the weight achieved is only kept. Although this phase should be regarded as a lifelong diet, it is rather discouraged due to the high proportion of animal fats and the associated health risks and consequential damages.

WHAT DIFFERENTIATES LCHF FROM ATKINS?

LCHF and Atkins are similar. Both largely refrain from carbohydrates as an energy source and are suitable for weight loss or the basic diet.

The Atkins diet is often linked to pure consumption of meat and fat. That is not right. Because only in the entry phase, the four-stage Atkins diet contains a lot of protein and fat, in the other diet phases, however, increasingly more carbohydrates from vegetables, berries, fruits and (whole grain) cereals.

LCHF sees the person

LCHF or Low Carb High Fat is less dogmatic and sees every person individually. Each body reacts differently to the intake of carbohydrates, and the health conditions play a significant role in the acceptance of carbohydrates. So there are LCHFler who consume only 5 grams of carbs daily, but others 30-50 grams and more.

Instead of carbohydrates, however, all natural fats (saturated fatty acids) occur, which should preferably be of animal origin. However, protein or protein should meet LCHF's requirements and should not be consumed excessively.

However, one principle distinguishes LCHF significantly from the Atkins diet

LCHF attaches great importance to a natural and good diet. This means that no industrially processed foods are on the menu, as well as poorly produced foods. This is especially true for animal products. Ecologically and regionally produced goods should always be given preference, if possible.

Meanwhile, the original idea of the Atkins diet has developed into a huge business that offers dietary supplements, protein shakes and bars, just to name a few products that would never be present in a classic LCHF diet.

THE FAQ ON ATKINS DIET

Does your body need carbohydrates?

To be precise; the body, especially the brains, do not need carbs but glucose. Glucose is released during the digestion of carbohydrates. The glucose is therefore used as energy. When you eat a lot of carbohydrates, the glucose is stored in the liver and muscles, so you always have a supply of glucose in your body.

When there is a surplus of glucose because you eat too many carbohydrates, it is stored in the form of fat.

In recent decades we have started to eat a lot more carbohydrates. We can easily handle much less.

What are net carbohydrates?

Net carbohydrates (net carbs) is a term used exclusively with Atkins products. This is because of the sweeteners needed to make the products tasty. These sweeteners replace the sugar.

These sweeteners, the polyols, must be officially listed as carbohydrates but do not work as carbohydrates. Your blood sugar hardly rises, if at all. That's why Atkins doesn't count them as carbohydrate, and you can deduct them from the total. Atkins has already done this for you, and therefore the net carbohydrates (net carbs) are stated on the packaging of the Atkins products that contain polyols.

This sum only applies to products that contain these substances, and there aren't that many. For all other products that you buy in the supermarket, you can simply count the number of carbohydrates listed in the nutritional value.

How should you count carbohydrates?

Eating fewer carbohydrates should not be too complicated; you want to last a long time. That is why it is best to count as little as possible.

By counting only carbohydrates, you do not have to count the rest (calories, proteins, fats).

You count carbohydrates by adding together the number of carbohydrates per product you eat. For the Atkins products, you count the net carbohydrates, and for all other foods, it applies that the carbohydrates are stated in the nutrition declaration on the label.

If the values are not listed, you can look up your carbohydrates on our carbohydrate counter or another database.

Does your body need fats?

By eating fewer carbohydrates, you eat more protein and also more fats. The words 'bold' and 'unhealthy' seem inextricably linked. The whole premise of eating less fat is based on simplistic ideas that we now know are incorrect.

First of all, the fat that you eat is not the fat that comes directly into the blood. Our liver determines the fat content in our blood for the most part. Liver function can be positively influenced by eating fewer carbohydrates.

The second point is the fat hypothesis. This says that the amount of cholesterol in your blood determines the chance of cardiovascular disease. Even now, after decades of research and years of low-fat advice, this statement has not been proven.

On average, less (saturated) fat is eaten, but the number of cardiovascular diseases has not decreased as a result. There is convincing scientific evidence that diets with fewer carbohydrates, as opposed to eating less fat, is positive in preventing cardiovascular disease, for example.

How many fats can you eat per day?

The same applies to fats and proteins and calories; you don't have to count them. Like proteins, fat causes saturation. Do not be afraid of using fat; you will never eat more of it than you like. It regulates itself. This does not mean that you can eat unlimited fat. However, when you eat fewer carbohydrates, you will notice that you are saturated faster.

When it comes to fats, choose the full products, i.e., full cheese, whole milk, and yogurt or Greek yogurt. Also choose from all types of meat and meat products such as bacon, sausage, and minced meat and not only for the lean types.

How many proteins can you eat per day?

When you count carbohydrates, you don't have to count proteins. Proteins are important with a low carbohydrate diet. Proteins are important for building materials and satiety. By eating enough protein, you will experience less appetite. Eat a protein-rich product every meal. Choose from meat, fish, chicken, egg, or cheese.

How many calories can you eat per day?

Do not count calories. Research shows that people who watch carbohydrates barely get more calories than those who are busy counting calories. Because of the protein and fat-rich diet, you are more saturated and will not eat more than you can eat.

Can you drink alcohol during Atkins?

Once in the fat burning process, the use of alcohol is a real 'game breaker.' The body will immediately use alcohol as energy, which will stop fat burning. Despite the sometimes low number of carbohydrates, wine and beer are the alcohol that cannot easily be combined with the Atkins diet.

Once you have reached your weight, you can, of course, experiment how much you can drink without gaining weight.

Can you follow Atkins if you don't eat meat?

That is certainly possible and requires a little more creativity. The recommendation is then to start in phase 2 with, for example, 30-35 grams of carbohydrates per day. In phase 2, you have a little more variety, and you can add nuts, seeds, and dairy to your diet.

Can you follow Atkins if you are vegan?

For vegans, Atkins is a bigger challenge, but it is not impossible. The proteins will have to come from seeds, nuts, soy products, soy and rice cheese, seitan, legumes and protein-rich grains such as quinoa. Due to the higher carbohydrate content, it may take a little longer before you lose weight. Start with 50 grams of carbohydrates per day.

What should you do if you no longer lose weight?

There is always time for everyone when things are not going so fast or for a while. Rest assured, this is part of it. Mainly be patient. Also, there are some other tips to help you through this period:

Drink enough. Drink 2 liters of total fluid per day. This can be water/coffee/ tea / light soft drinks and lemonade without sugar.

Provide two servings of vegetables per day. In phase 1, these are, for example, spinach, lettuce, and endive. Eat a portion of 150 grams of vegetables or 50 grams of lettuce per meal, so vegetables for lunch and dinner.

Make sure you have enough fat. Do not eat everything lean or 0% fat. When eating low carbohydrates, you need fat as fuel.

Make sure you have enough protein per meal. Just eating lettuce at lunch is not enough. This should include something of chicken/fish/ meat or egg.

Avoid alcohol in the first stages; alcohol influences fat burning.

Feel free to use Atkins products but stick to 1 bar per day when it comes to snacks.

Make sure you do not eat hidden carbohydrates. Look on the packaging with the ingredients to see if it doesn't contain a lot of sugar. Sauces, for example, quite often contain a lot of sugars.

Measure your waist circumference. Sometimes you do not lose weight in kilos but centimeters.

What should you do when you arrive again?

A weight fluctuation of 1-2 kilos is normal. If you gain more than 2 kilos, try to eat 10 grams fewer carbohydrates per day and keep an exact record of what you eat.

Of course, you can also choose to go to phase 1 or phase 2 again for 1 or 2 weeks. That way, you will automatically return to the correct rhythm.

Can you eat out during Atkins?

A low carb diet like Atkins can easily be combined with eating out. Whether you like shish kebab or sushi, chicken or steak, every restaurant or even fast food chains offer options for low carbohydrate eating.

What do you choose?

- All types of chicken, meat or fish with gravy and sauces (without sugar)
- Stews without potatoes
- Grilled fish and shellfish
- Gyros, lamb

- Roasted vegetables
- All types of salads without pasta and potatoes
- Bouillon
- Carpaccio
- Onion soup
- Bourgingon beef

And what better way to leave it:

- Pasta, risotto
- Garlic bread, baguette
- Chips, nachos
- Quiches
- Potato soup
- Fries
- Fried potatoes, mashed potatoes
- Noodles, rice, fried rice

Can you follow Atkins during pregnancy or while breastfeeding?

If you are pregnant or breastfeeding, losing weight is not recommended. Eating less fast sugars and carbohydrates are, of course, always healthy. In this phase choose lots of vegetables, salads, whole grains and cereal products, sufficient dairy (proteins), fruit and legumes.

Can you follow Atkins if you use medication?

Healthy food is always preferable to unhealthy food. Even if you use medication, some medicines can influence the pace of weight loss. Always consult with your doctor, practice assistant, or dietician when you change your lifestyle. Even if you have lost a lot of weight, it is advisable to evaluate the use of medication regularly.

What types of flour can I use to replace normal flour?

If you require eating lesser carbohydrates, you will discover that especially the products that contain starch and flour contain a lot of carbohydrates. Unfortunately, when baking food yourself, you cannot simply omit the flour or flour. Many people replace the flour with almond flour and coconut flour. Feel free to experiment with this, the dish may look different but taste good. It also pays to search the internet or in books for low-carbohydrate dishes. Many enthusiastic cooking enthusiasts are happy to share their experiences.

In which way do the Atkins products fit into the diet?

The Atkins range consists of meal components such as carbohydrate-reduced bread, crackers, muesli, and pasta. Also, there is a large choice of snacks and shakes.

The reduced carbohydrate products from Atkins can replace products with normally a lot of carbohydrates. This way, you can easily eat fewer carbohydrates by choosing the Atkins bread, the crackers and replacing the pasta with Atkins pasta every day.

Snacks from Atkins are low in carbohydrates and fit well into any low carbohydrate diet. You can choose from bars, and ready-to-drink shakes.

Because the products are not vitaminized, they are not mealed replacements. If you still want to use an Atkins product as a meal replacement, make sure you eat enough fiber from vegetables or raw vegetables elsewhere in the day.

Which sweeteners are used in the products?

Atkins is the best taste with fewer carbohydrates. We choose the ingredients that ensure the best taste and structure. This also applies to sweeteners. For this reason, all types of sweeteners and sugar substitutes are used that best suit a product.

Sweeteners may appear to be in the dark; they have been extensively researched and approved and offer a good alternative to sugar in our products.

The Atkins 'Lowered in carbohydrates' bread consists of the most of wheat. How can it be low in carbohydrate?

It is true that the bread consists largely of wheat. However, it is the different types of wheat grain in the lowered carbohydrate bread that make the difference. A large part of the wheat that we add consists of wheat gluten, wheat fibers, and wheat bran. Wheat gluten is proteins and therefore, do not provide carbohydrates. The wheat fibers and wheat bran are indigestible fibers. These are useful ingredients but do not belong to the carbohydrates. This is how our bread is 'reduced in carbohydrates.'

Are the Atkins products meal replacements or intended as a snack?

The principle of Atkins is that you can eat 3 meals a day with several snacks as desired. The Atkins products are therefore not made as a meal replacement. The products are also not vitaminized, a requirement to be called a meal replacement. We see many people using the Atkins products for breakfast or lunch. If you eat enough proteins, fiber, vegetables and healthy fats for the rest of the day, it makes no difference when you eat something, and you can plan meals in a way that suits you best.

Are the Atkins products suitable for everyone? Also, for children and the elderly

Everyone can eat fewer carbohydrates to promote a healthy lifestyle. The Atkins products contain more proteins and fibers and fewer sugars. This makes them healthy products that everyone can use. Some people may suffer from the sweeteners (polyols) that replace the sugars in some Atkins bars. To do this, look at the entry list and the nutritional values on the package. The sweeteners, which also occur in other sugar-free products, can sometimes cause intestinal complaints in the beginning. For those who have these complaints, it is advisable to start with small quantities so that you will have no or fewer problems with this.

CONCLUSION

The Atkins Diet is not for everyone, that's for sure. But it can be quite successful if you bring discipline and are ready to say goodbye to sugar and carbohydrates. A waiver in this direction is certainly not unhealthy however, you should check yourself for safety regularly medical check if you pull through the diet phases over several months.

Because ultimately you force your body with the ketosis first in a hunger metabolism, which is not intended as a standard. The longer you stay in this unnatural state, the more important it is to keep your health in view by the professional.

While the Atkins Diet is a successful way to lose weight quickly, it should not be a long-term change in diet. With too much fat and protein and too few vegetables, fruits and fiber, this strict low carb diet is anything but balanced and therefore not suitable for a permanent diet. Too high is the risk of health damage and dysfunction.

The Atkins Diet is only suitable for rapid weight loss and as a short-term diet. However, if you are looking for a diet that is also suitable in the longer term, should opt for a diet with a moderate amount of carbohydrates in combination with lots of fresh fiber-rich fruits and vegetables, which is easier to maintain in the long run. Also, vegetable fats such as olive oil should be preferred to animal fats.

Made in the
USA
Middletown, DE